RAPID WEIGHT LOSS HYPNOSIS

2 BOOKS IN 1: HYPNOTIC GASTRIC BAND & POSITIVE AFFIRMATIONS FOR WEIGHT LOSS. STOP COMPULSIVE EATING AND STOP SUGAR CRAVING WITH SELF-HYPNOSIS AND GUIDED MEDITATION

MARTIN ELAND

TABLE OF CONTENTS

Hypnotic Gastric Band

Stop emotional eating and lose weight quickly with self-hypnosis. Improve your lifestyle and develop healthy habits to feel more confident and happy with yourself.

By:Martin Eland

INTRODUCTION

Gastric band hypnotherapy is a technique utilized to propose to the subliminal that you've had a gastric band fitted around your stomach to help you lose weight.

Thought about a final retreat, gastric band surgery includes fitting a band around the upper part of the stomach. This confines the measure of food you can physically eat, empowering weight loss. It's a surgical procedure, and along these lines accompanies possible dangers and difficulties.

Gastric band hypnotherapy or having a 'virtual gastric band' fitted doesn't require surgery. It is a technique utilized by hypnotherapists to get the inner mind to accept there's been a gastric band fitted. On an oblivious level, you will accept that you've had the physical procedure and that your stomach has decreased in size.

The process doesn't include surgery or prescription and is completely safe.

Gastric band hypnosis refers to a hypnosis treatment for weight loss. This treatment is sometimes additionally referred to as 'Hypno gastric band,' 'virtual gastric band,' or 'gastric band surgery hypnosis.'

What is Gastric Band Hypnotherapy?

Gastric band hypnotherapy is a ground-breaking, intriguing program that persuades your inner mind that your stomach is now full, although, in reality, the portion size was little.

The virtual gastric band offers a specific option in contrast to an expensive surgery, which, similar to every clinical intercession, accompanies hazards just as expected advantages.

Who is Gastric Band Hypnosis Suitable for?

As a rule, I would propose that gastric band hypnosis is a perfect part of a hypnosis weight loss program for somebody who:

Has something other than a couple of pounds to be hydrated

Recognizes as being on the emotional eating side of the range

Gastric band hypnosis is the 'substantial weapons' methodology in the arrangement of a weight loss trance specialist.

There is nothing that blocks somebody with a mindful

eating issue to remember the virtual gastric band for their weight loss program. If you feel attracted to gastric band hypnosis, it might be the perfect thing for you.

What Does the Gastric Band Hypnosis Treatment Involve?

Like some other hypnosis program, gastric band hypnosis begins with a profound unwinding convention that makes you as relaxed as conceivable both physically and intellectually.

When you are profoundly relaxed, the trance inducer will utilize an incredible content based on the suggestion that professes to your inner mind that you are experiencing gastric detour surgery.

The fundamental hidden idea here is that the inner mind doesn't have the foggiest idea about the difference between reality and a creative mind. If you can persuade your inner mind that you can accomplish something, at that point, your psyche mind will convey success.

To persuade your inner mind, your subliminal specialist may even utilize scents and sounds you would connect with an emergency clinic setting. This will be joined with embedding ground-breaking post-hypnotic suggestions such that, starting now and into the foreseeable future, your stomach might have the option to eat little portions.

Initially, gastric band hypnosis utilized alone in a once-off session may not be sufficient to help you beat your weight issue. It is greatly improved utilized as a part of an exhaustive weight loss hypnosis program, which tends to all parts of your weight issue such that it's customized for you as a person.

The virtual gastric detour surgery will be acted in a hypnotic stupor state with the goal that the suggestions will sink into your inner mind. If they sink in even only a little piece, your psyche mind will assist you with losing weight by guiding you towards eating littler portions.

Try not to expect that your conscious mind will be persuaded that you have experienced surgery. It won't be. It doesn't need to be. That isn't what makes a difference in the process.

Rather, change your mindset and desires to take a gander at the virtual gastric band as an apparatus, as an unfortunate chore. What makes a difference are the impacts of the treatment on the psyche mind and the changes you make to your eating regimen post-treatment.

When you receive this down to a business mindset, you are better prepared to get the best out of your treatment because you won't get derailed your mind's inbuilt blue pencils 'assessing' how realistic the session was for you.

A gastric band is an adjustable silicone gadget utilized in weight loss surgery. The band is set around the upper segment of the stomach to make a little pocket over the gadget. This confines the measure of food that can be put away in the stomach, making it difficult to eat enormous sums.

The point of a gastric band is to limit the measure of food an individual can physically eat, making them feel full in the wake of eating next to no to support weight loss. For a great many people who have this surgery, it is a final retreat after attempting different strategies for weight loss. Like any surgery, fitting a gastric band accompanies dangers.

Gastric band hypnosis

Gastric band hypnosis can help people with losing weight, without the dangers that accompany surgery. Numerous hypnotherapists utilize a two-dimensional methodology. First, they hope to identify the main driver of your emotional eating.

Utilizing hypnosis, the therapist can urge you to recollect since a long time ago overlooked encounters encompassing food that might be subliminally influencing you now. Tending to and perceiving any unhealthy thought designs encompassing food can be useful before completing gastric band hypnotherapy.

Next, the hypnotherapist will do the virtual gastric band treatment. The procedure is intended to propose, at a subconscious mind level, that you have had an activity to embed a gastric band. The point is for your body to react to this suggestion by making you feel faster, as though you had the real surgery.

Hypnotherapists clarify why diets don't work for weight loss

Many eating regimen plans are transitory and can be difficult to keep up on an on-going premise, frequently because they are excessively prohibitive, or they absolutely deny us of our preferred foods.

These systems can be held on to the present moment yet don't work so well over the long haul. Making us tally calories or deliberately measure portion sizes or even absolutely overlooking sorts of foods, numerous weight control plans can make us increasingly fixated on food and eating. This can remove the joy from eating and lead us to long for a greater amount of specific foods, and an eating routine gorge/gorge cycle can begin.

How gastric band hypnosis works

Utilizing unwinding techniques, a hypnotherapist will place you into a state of hypnosis. In this relaxed state, your psyche is increasingly open to suggestions. Now hypnotherapists make suggestions to your inner mind. With gastric band hypnotherapy, this suggestion is that you've had a physical band fitted.

The mind is ground-breaking, so if your subliminal acknowledges these suggestions, your behavior will change in like manner. As a rule, alongside the 'fitting' of the virtual gastric band, suggestions encompassing certainty and behavior will be made to assist you with focusing on this change in lifestyle.

Numerous therapists will likewise show self-hypnosis techniques so you can upgrade the work you've done after the session. Instructing yourself on nourishment and exercise is regularly exhorted, too, to advance physical wellbeing and prosperity.

The procedure

Your first gathering with the hypnotherapist will probably be an underlying counsel where you talk about what you plan to gain from hypnotherapy. This is a chance to discuss any past weight loss endeavors, your eating habits, any medical problems, and your general disposition towards food. This information will give the therapist a clearer idea of what will help and whether some other types of treatment should be considered.

The procedure itself is intended to mirror gastric band surgery and enable your inner mind to trust it has really occurred. To make the experience progressively legitimate, numerous hypnotherapists will incorporate the sounds and scents of an operating theater. Your therapist will start by bringing you into a profoundly relaxed state, otherwise called hypnosis. You will know about what's going on and will be in control consistently.

When you are in a hypnotic state, the therapist will talk you through the activity. They will clarify bit by bit what occurs in surgery, from being put under the sedative, to making the principal entry point, fitting the band itself, and sewing up the cut. Sounds and scents of an operating performance center will upgrade the experience, to convince your subliminal that what's being said is really transpiring.

As recently referenced, different suggestions might be incorporated during the procedure to expand fearlessness. When the procedure is finished, your hypnotherapist may show you some self-hypnosis techniques to assist you with remaining on target at home.

Some hypnotherapists will demand that you return for follow-up arrangements to screen the virtual band's success and to make any alterations. This happens when people get the physical band fitted as well. For a few, it very well may be useful to proceed with hypnotherapy sessions as part of a drawn-out weight the executive's plan. This permits the hypnotherapist to work with you to address fundamental issues encompassing food and confidence.

Gastric band hypnosis should shape part of weight the board program that tends to sustenance and exercise habits. It is the mix of changing habits in both body and mind that is regularly best for those looking for weight loss.

By what method will I feel after?

The general point of gastric band hypnosis is to energize a more advantageous relationship with food. At the point when your inner mind trusts you have had a gastric band fitted, it will accept your stomach is littler. This, thus, causes your cerebrum to convey messages that you are full subsequent to devouring less food.

For the individuals who indulge, perceiving when you're physically full can be difficult. Sometimes we eat only for the taste (or solace), overlooking whether we are physically eager. Figuring out how to perceive the physical vibes of being hungry and full is useful for developing healthy eating habits.

In contrast to gastric band surgery, the virtual gastric band doesn't have any physical reactions. For a few, real surgery can cause queasiness, retching, and heartburn. As gastric band hypnosis is certainly not a physical process, it won't cause side effects this way.

The procedure ought to be a charming and loosening up understanding, with a great many people detailing a feeling of quiet when they come out of hypnosis.

Will it work for me?

A typical inquiry for that difficult hypnotherapy is - will it work for me? Lamentably, it is anything but a straightforward instance of yes or no; it is generally up to you. Hypnotherapy helps people with a scope of concerns, but is particularly valuable with regards to evolving habits. Consequently, it is regularly successful in helping people create healthy eating habits and lose weight. Much the same as some other weight loss framework, it will require your absolute responsibility.

You are bound to get what you need from gastric band hypnotherapy if you have confidence in the process and your therapist. Being agreeable and believing your hypnotherapist is basic. This is the reason it is exhorted that you set aside an effort to explore hypnotherapists in your general vicinity and discover progressively about them, how they work, and what their qualifications involve. You can mastermind to meet with them before the procedure to guarantee you feel great with them.

If you are focused on making a lifestyle change, have confidence in the procedure, and trust your hypnotherapist, gastric band hypnosis should work for you.

CHAPTER ONE: HYPNOTIC GASTRIC BAND SCRIPTS

Free hypnotherapy content can be utilized by a prepared therapist or by a person who needs to lose weight and with a smidgen of preparing in self-hypnosis.

People – Self-hypnosis. To incite a state of light stupor, lie or plunk down someplace agreeable and with least unsettling influence. Close your eyes and hinder your relaxing. As you hinder your breathing, start to physically unwind from the highest point of your head down to your toes. This can take anyplace somewhere in the range of 5 and 15 minutes.

At that point, gradually tally yourself down from 10 to 1. In this relaxed state, you would then be able to open your eyes and gradually read through this hypnotherapy content. You can, if you wish, change the language structure if you are doing self-hypnosis, for example, "every one of my feelings is acceptable, every one of my feelings is there for a reason," and so forth, anyway this isn't carefully vital as your oblivious mind will see paying little heed to the punctuation tense.

When you have finished it, you can check yourself back to full conscious mindfulness, tallying up from 1 to 10.

Rehash every day and screen your advancement.

"The entirety of your feelings is acceptable." The entirety of your feelings is there for a reason. There is no difference between the five external detects, contact, taste, sight, smell, and hearing, and the entirety of your internal faculties that we call feelings. They are there to support you and guide you, so you can deal with yourself in a manner that is generally useful to you.

Your feelings resemble the measures and lights on the leading scramble group of a vehicle. These lights and measures on the vehicle are there for a reason. They help you to realize what to do to keep it running effectively with the goal that it will run dependably for quite a while. This permits you to take advantage of your responsibility for the vehicle—the best execution and worth. The equivalent goes for you and your body; feelings help reveal to you how to take the best consideration of yourself.

If you rewarded a vehicle for the way you have been treating your body, the vehicle would before long be in a tough situation, similarly that you are in a tough situation now. At the point when the oil light illuminates in a vehicle, the driver doesn't maneuver into a gas station and put more petroleum into the tank, particularly if the tank is as of now full. This is the thing that you have never been helping to body.

You are here because, in the past, when you felt a

feeling, for example, uneasiness, dissatisfaction, weariness, discouragement, or whatever, and you have attempted to take care of that feeling. You realize this is valid because you have attempted it, and it didn't work.

At the point when the oil light on a vehicle goes on, it shows that the driver needs to check the oil.

At the point when the temperature light goes on, the driver needs to check the water in the radiator.

At the point when the breeze shield wiper liquid light goes on, the driver needs to place in increasingly liquid, etc. These lights are acceptable. They should be gone as well. Placing more petroleum in the vehicle won't help any of these circumstances.

At the point when you feel on edge, it is a sign to glance around, something in your life needs fixing.

At the point when you feel discouraged, it is a sign to turn out to be progressively successful. It's a source of inspiration.

At the point when you feel frustrated, it is a sign what you are doing isn't working, have a go at something else.

At the point when you focus, it implies that you are attempting to do excessively to make everything great.

At the point when you feel forlornness, it implies that you have a healthy want for human contact. Call somebody, compose a letter, check your email, join a club, or become a volunteer.

Eating doesn't fulfill any of these feelings, anything else than placing more petroleum in your vehicle will fix an oil or temperature issue.

Presently you will think that it's simpler to comprehend what every one of your feelings is attempting to show for you to do. I suggest that you invest some energy after you go home and record a portion of the feelings that have "caused" you to eat before. At that point record, what that feeling really implies. For instance, sorrow implies that I am feeling insufficient, defenseless, or miserable. The correct activity is to take a gander at my life and identify the zone or zones where I feel along these lines. At that point, start to build up a strategy to begin to make things different. At long last, start working on the arrangement. At that point, watch as your downturn blurs away.

As you would now be able to see, the entirety of your feelings is acceptable. Similarly, tantamount to the five detects. They are there to control you. Someplace you got the wires crossed. Presently we are rectifying that.

The reason your wires may have gotten crossed is that some time back, most likely, when you were extremely youthful, you felt a feeling, and you were unable to act in light of it. You had the feeling, however, attempt as you may, and because of your conditions, could do close to nothing or nothing about what was causing the feeling.

So even if you understood what the feeling was attempting to let you know, there was little you could do about it. You ended up overlooking what the feeling even implied for you to do. You, at that point, erroneously discovered impermanent solace in the interruption of food. It didn't help. In any case, there was more food and more feelings, and you fell into that trench. Presently you are moving out of that trench.

You are currently prepared to start a life that is substantially more fulfilling than the one you have been living. Presently you are fit for fulfilling yourself more than ever.

Presently, when a feeling comes up again, you'll comprehend what to do. You will start to anticipate following up on your feelings in a more fulfilling way. For instance, if you feel desolate, you can call a companion, visit somebody, or go to a spot where you can meet people. Forlornness can never be happy with the food. You currently comprehend that to be a reality.

What's more, just as dejection can't be fulfilled by food, neither can pressure, disappointment, nervousness, sadness, weariness, or some other feeling.

You are currently liberated from the baffling cycle that has caused you so much misery and weight gain. From this time ahead, you will eat just when you are certain that you need re-filling. You will currently start to fulfill yourself in numerous new and more intriguing and satisfying ways.

Beginning now and into the foreseeable future, when you get a feeling, and it isn't hunger, you will essentially say, STOP, this is significant, I'm giving this my 100% exertion. My feelings are attempting to disclose to me something significant. At that point, tune in to the feeling and start to follow up on it".

CHAPTER TWO: HOW GASTRIC BAND HYPNOTHERAPY WORKS

Envision feeling like you've recently experienced gastric band surgery, everything from the sedation to the surgical procedure and recuperation while never going to a medical clinic.

That is the thing that gastric band hypnotherapy does. It makes the whole setting for gastric band surgery, utilizing hypnotherapy performed by an authorized gastric banding expert and at-home hypnosis guided by a sound tape.

The process is a huge number of dollars less expensive, contains no physical hazard, and causes the client to feel that their stomach size has contracted significantly, making them settle on improved choices about portion sizes at dinner times.

Gastric band hypnotherapy has a sure success rate; however, it's anything but an enchantment pill for weight loss. Similarly, as surgery makes the state important to assist you with settling on better choices, you should, in reality, at that point cause them for change to happen. Thus it is with hypnosis.

There has been a significant flood in the volume of people being clinically determined to have heftiness, and various arrangements have been considered to assist them with diminishing weight. Yet, many weight loss diet programs neglect to convey lasting results if, so far as that is concerned, they work by any means. Slims down are regularly just followed for a brief timeframe, and any weight loss accomplished is returned soon a while later.

Gastric band surgeries are expensive and contain many threats for the person. Likewise, there are sometimes undesirable impacts, for example, inside anomaly, feeling wiped out and really being wiped out.

As an elective choice, it is currently felt that gastric band hypnotherapy assists with getting comparable results by ingraining the conviction that the stomach limit is drastically decreased when no physical change has been made. A hypnotic methodology works by adjusting an individual's musings. Gainful recommendations made while in hypnosis can have lasting results.

To accomplish life-long positive considerations and feelings about food and eating conduct, gastric band hypnotherapy may help to securely and successfully animate weight loss and forestall over-utilization. Extraordinary results have been created with contextual investigation clients who have had gastric band hypnosis. They've eaten decreased servings even though they have never had gastric band surgery.

The procedure involves a concise course of medicines that lead up to virtual gastric band surgery happening while you are in a trance. Virtual fragrances and furthermore clamors will regularly be utilized to imitate the medical clinic setting before the client is brought once again from this trance-like state. The aim is for the person to see on a psyche level that they've really had a physical surgery and subsequently accept that lone reasonable portions of food can be eaten. "Gastric band hypnotherapy is practical and hazard free contrasted with the significant expense of surgery and the potential for difficulties."

In one investigation, the subject shed more than 3 kilos in only 10 days and kept thinning down as the months passed by. It is conceivable to return for hypnotherapy to have the band modified or sometimes removed to accomplish the ideal weight.

The subliminal specialist may assist the individual in changing their patterns, going ahead to keep up their new eating conduct. Gastric band hypnosis is hence a perfect trade for an unsavory careful treatment, with no of the dangers and issues that can regularly occur.

WHAT SHOULD I LOOK FOR IN A THERAPIST?

Numerous specialists that practice gastric band hypnosis are knowledgeable in practice. Some will lead with this as their primary zone of specialism, as others lead with relieving smoking. Be that as it may, when it comes to what to search for in an advisor, my primary concerns would be:

Check for a long history of success, search for any letters, grants, and tributes on free audit destinations.

Ensure you are OK with the advisor, I've heard reports of people not finishing courses of treatment because something about the specialists' style sometimes falls short for them. Manner of speaking and so forth.

WHY IT'S MORE THAN HYPNOTHERAPY

Keep in mind, when losing weight, don't persuade yourself that your "support" is your hero. You can't lose weight by saying a particular something and doing another at that point reprimanding your prop for coming up short.

Hypnotherapy is the perfect help for an individual goal of losing weight. Yet, it can likewise help with portion control, cheap food aversion, and numerous different things intended to bolster you through the procedure subconsciously.

Those plans on losing weight will have the best success; however, eating less isn't great. Particularly those who expect you to buy shakes and powders as that is a prop. What you truly need is a lifestyle change, and an NLP prepared trance specialist will assist you with making gastric band hypnosis work for you.

The most effective method to CONTINUE YOUR SUCCESS

Proceeded with the success of your gastric band hypnotherapy sessions is exacerbated by finishing the recommended number of sessions. You can see extraordinary results in a couple of sessions, yet you should consistently like any type of prescription or therapy to complete the number of sessions your specialist proposed.

Gastric Band Hypnotherapy causes you to stop habitual over-eating conduct, which has prompted weight gain, just as resolve the oblivious explanations behind long term over-eating. We are entirely brought into the world with the sense to eat when we are eager and stop when we are fulfilled, which implies that our vitality and wholesome needs are met while keeping up a healthy weight. In any case, a significant number of us lose touch with that impulse during youth when we were urged to disregard our body's signs and eat everything on the plate, just as being supported or rewarded with food even though we aren't ravenous. What's more, "starting to eat better" makes a negative pattern of hardship thinking and afterward, over-eating conduct. Sugar-rich nibble foods can prompt sugar enslavement and over-eating, and the broadly held yet incorrect conviction that we ought to eat at regular intervals to abstain from getting ravenous implies that we lose touch with the impulses that are normal to us and that are intended to guarantee we are a healthy weight.

Gastric band hypnotherapy utilizes both hypnotherapy and neuro-linguistic programming (NLP) strategies to persuade people that they have had a gastric band fitted. Real 'gastric band' surgery includes precisely limiting the stomach's ability. This decreased stomach limit implies that the feeling of totality becomes evident considerably more rapidly, and the measure of food expended is subsequently diminished. Gastric band hypnotherapy can prompt the entirety of the advantages of gastric band surgery yet without the feelings of trepidation, dangers, cost, and symptoms of experiencing real surgery.

The gastric band hypnotherapy includes profound unwinding during which you will be guided through the whole activity in your creative mind, bit by bit, from an organization of the sedative, to the first cut to the closing of the entry point. Before long, you should feel the impression of completion after only a couple of significant pieces, which implies you will feel less eager, less regularly, and eat less when you do eat.

The therapy includes different procedures, for example, positive proposal, representation, and NLP. At the Curative Hypnotherapy Clinic, we will likewise utilize diagnostic hypnotherapy to identify and resolve the oblivious underlying driver of the over-eating that has prompted the weight gain with the goal that you can accomplish and keep up a healthy weight for the remainder of your life.

Being over-weight is a result of expending a higher number of calories than your body needs in terms of the vitality that it employs. As a rule, eating even though you are not eager and proceeding to eat in any event when you are fulfilled is the fundamental driver of weight gain. Furthermore, eating a lot of those foods that are calorie thick, for example, food and beverages that are high in sugar, likewise add to weight gain.

You are generally over-eating when:

You don't bite your food entirely and hence eat rapidly. As a result, you don't see your body's signs revealing to you that you have eaten enough food and the taste buds in your mouth have not been completely fulfilled, which prompts needing "something decent" in the wake of completing a meal.

You deliberately disregard the sign that you are fulfilled and keep eating.

You eat when you are not genuinely hungry yet exhausted or pushed or feel a "need" to eat; regularly, this implies nibble food between your meals.

Gastric Band Hypnotherapy needs to be joined by our Analytical Hypnotherapy methods to identify and, for all time, settle the underlying driver of the over-eating.

CHAPTER THREE: TYPES OF GASTRIC BANDING

A type of bariatric surgery that decreases the size of your stomach by utilizing a silicone band is known as Adjustable Gastric Band (AGB) surgery. Weight loss happens since your littler stomach can't hold as much food. After some time, the measure of weight you lose is controlled by your primary care physician who alters the band, either fixing or releasing it to take into consideration an expansion or diminishing in weight loss. There is an assortment of bands used to achieve this, and it is essential to learn as much as possible about them before choosing with your PCP, which is the best for you.

Created in 1984 by Professor Dag Hallberg, the Swedish band was the first known adjustable gastric band, as per the specialists at Obesity Surgery. By 1985, he got his patent, anyway, it was just accessible in Sweden, Denmark, and Norway. As indicated by the specialists at Weight Loss Surgery, it opened up worldwide in 1996. The Swedish band works by isolating your stomach into two segments by setting the band around the highest segment of your stomach, as is valid for most AGBs. It either permits more food or less food to enter your lower stomach as required by being fixed or disengaged as required. You, at last, lose less weight since the upper portion of the stomach tops off with food rapidly before going through, you feeling satisfied sooner, which encourages you to eat less. The inflatable used to make these alterations lines the whole band, making the band more adaptable for this procedure than some different bands available.

Not long after Professor Hallberg got his Swedish patent for the band, Lubomir Kuzmak, an American specialist, planned what has gotten named as the Lap-Band. Dr. Kuzmak utilized for his patent in 1985, as indicated by Obesity Surgery. The difference anyway was that not normal for Professor Hallberg, Kuzmak's patent was for the United States as it were. Although the Lap-Band has since been updated, it must be balanced at a limit of two millimeters initially, and in this manner, it was not entirely adaptable. It would now be able to be adjusted 7 to 8 millimeters. As indicated by the Lap-Band Guide, the Lap-Band has been utilized in Europe since 1993, despite its American patent.

In 2001, it got FDA endorsement to be utilized in the United States. Around the world, in excess of 350,000 Lap-Band techniques have since been performed.

After the structure and patent of the Lap-Band, the Midband was planned by Dr. Vincent Frering in Lyon, France. This band is innately different in structure from the Swedish Band and the Lap-Band. It has a bigger inflatable and is somewhat shorter. Having had involvement in both the Swedish and Lap-Bands, Dr. Frering planned the Midband as such to give a milder framework. This assists with guaranteeing that the band doesn't aggravate the covering of the gastric divider, which forestalls disintegration and disturbance of the band from happening. What's more, the Midband doesn't have sharp edges as a portion of its counterparts do, and it is effortlessly identified by X-beams, removing the mystery from modifications.

The Easyband is the most current expansion to the gastric-band family and works like none other. The Easyband is simply innovative. It doesn't require a saline answer for flattening or expansion during alterations of the inflatable. Inside the band is an engine and a microchip. At the point when the time has come to modify your band, the specialist will utilize a handheld gadget looking like a remote control to find the chip. When found, he will impart a sign to the chip, which advises the band to relax or fix. It must be noticed that the Easyband is as yet trial, and there is at present no proof to demonstrate or scatter its adequacy.

CHAPTER FOUR: TECHNIQUES USED IN HYPNOTHERAPY FOR WEIGHT LOSS

Hypnosis occurs in all therapy.

One attribute of the hypnotic state is deliberation. I mean genuinely being in one spot, but mentally being in another.

This happens to a significant degree when we dream around evening time. Genuinely you're sleeping, yet mentally you're elsewhere.

Fish asking what water is

Think about advising. The guide may view hypnosis as 'off limits region' for their discouraged client, even as they begin getting some information about their life and their past. In any case, when you ask a client inquiries identifying with real factors outside the therapy room, you are welcoming them to 'trance out.'

At the point when the client turns out to be more mentally checked out – state – the separation they experienced a year ago than to the right here/right now therapy room, at that point, the 'deliberation' component of trance is in full play.

The most popular methodology utilized in hypnotherapy is called Suggestion. The word in this setting has a comparative, yet not equal importance to that in regular use. 'Proposal' in hypnotherapy implies a thought given to the deeper part of your mind – the inner mind – to help change your reasoning with the goal that you are bound to practice consistently, eat more moderately, or whatever you are looking to accomplish. A recommendation can work all alone (promoting is one type of this); however, it turns out to be much increasingly ground-breaking when joined with hypnosis. There are numerous kinds of hypnotic recommendations, one of which is called a direct proposal: 'You presently permit yourself to value your qualities.' This is a clear solicitation that you think with a specific goal in mind. Sometimes, be that as it may, we may improve something increasingly unobtrusive: 'I wonder what number of people have thought beneficial things about you, yet never said?' This keeps away from an immediate solicitation and is along these lines called a backhanded proposal. Some proposal is a fantastic vehicle that drives you towards your goal. Believe it or not – there is an additional figurative proposal. Note in that sentence; we utilized the illustrations: 'amazing vehicle,' 'drive,' and 'goal.' You are no uncertainty mindful that extraordinary speakers frequently use allegory because of its strong capacity to pass on thoughts.

A few of the accompanying procedures originate from a quick change technique known as Neuro-linguistic Programming (NLP). They are valuable instruments all alone, yet become much progressively incredible when joined with hypnosis. 'Going about as though' When we try to roll out an improvement in our life, we are bound to be successful if we can do this in each appropriate manner. For example, if you wish to be a non-smoker, you should pretend that you have stopped smoking a long time ago. What's more, when you likewise talk, think, and feel like a non-smoker, it turns out to be such a great amount of simpler to stay free. At the point when utilized within hypnotherapy, this strategy can enable you 'to program' your mind to accomplish these far-reaching developments.

Demonstrating Similar to 'Going about as though'

Demonstrating includes our picking somebody we consider to be an extraordinarily good example – an incredible sportsperson, a gifted speaker, or whatever – and giving a valiant effort to be much the same as them. Modeling is that the more that we make ourselves like them; at that point, the simpler it is to accomplish what they do. Tying down In certain circumstances, we might want to 'switch on' specific feelings – tranquility, certainty, or whatever. Mooring empowers us to do this by connecting a basic activity or occasion to a time when we were in that helpful state. At that point, when we need to bring that creative state back, we can utilize the activity to inspire it again. Mindfulness When we concentrate our minds on something that exists as of now and do as such without making a decision about it, at that point, we're utilizing Mindfulness.

The advantages of rehearsing Mindfulness are significant, and we incorporate parts of it within huge numbers of our self-hypnosis chronicles. It improves our capacity to center, study, and work. Further, our typical programmed decisions control us less, helping us change our reasoning without any problem. For example, we can manage memory more effectively when we can pick our opinion of it. Inventive Visualization When joined with the intensity of hypnosis, imaginative representation can assist with creating quick and lasting change. Which is the reason we use it widely within our chronicles. When we picture something in our minds, the deeper part of the cerebrum can't differentiate between that picture and reality. So envisioning your business has gotten progressively successful, for example, will be acknowledged as evident by the inner mind. As a result, you will have a more prominent conviction that you can accomplish this result. Mental Rehearsal We can utilize the procedure of perception for another reason – to intellectually practice something. Again, the mind will react just as you truly were practicing; thus, you could, for example, envision rehearsing your golf, in this manner improving your genuine presentation.

Desensitization

Our mind sometimes figures out how to have unjustified feelings. Fears are a prime example – the cerebrum makes a connection between an item (an arachnid, for instance) and dread. Hypnotherapy can, be that as it may, help the mind break this association through a procedure called desensitization. This includes envisioning the item when quiet and permitting the mind to bit by bit, fix that dangerous learning. The Prediction Error Shift When you approach a circumstance, your mind will anticipate what may occur straightaway. If, for example, you have a dread of statures, as you stroll towards an extension, you will envision feeling on edge. Be that as it may, if you jump on the scaffold and feel quiet for reasons unknown, the cerebrum should conform to this reality. It will moderate its desires for future comparative occasions just somewhat, yet if this astounding smoothness continued happening, then your mind would hold shifting to where you would lose your dread. This is known as the Prediction Error Shift, and when utilized within a self-hypnosis recording, your mind can roll out this improvement easily and rapidly.

Cognitive Behavioral Therapy

Cognitive Behavioral Therapy (CBT) is a type of brain research that is extremely powerful in treating a wide scope of issues. It depends on the reason that our reasoning isn't generally perfect – about everybody makes emotional issues by this implies, however having found our own maverick musings, we can substitute increasingly accommodating ones. For example, we may disclose to ourselves that we should accomplish something, yet we truly mean we might want to. Rolling out that improvement can assuage a lot of worry in our lives.

CHAPTER FIVE: WHAT YOU NEED TO KNOW ABOUT HYPNOTIC GASTRIC BAND THERAPY

Gastric Band Hypnotherapy is a well-known option for those thinking about gastric band surgery. It's mainstream because it's totally protected and significantly more reasonable than different choices. With a success rate of over 90%, it's no big surprise that an ever-increasing number of people are going to the Virtual Gastric Band rather than the careful gastric band. Probably best of all, it tends to be done from the solace of one's own home.

This elective decision to surgery accommodates a lifestyle change that occurs without conscious exertion utilizing the intensity of the unconscious mind. You feel more joyful, lighter, increasingly enthusiastic, and progressively self-assured in a way that is often astounding. A "no exertion" weight, the executive's program sounds unrealistic. The thing is, it's not so much about the weight of the board. It's tied in with managing the reasons why we eat a lot in any case. Losing weight is only a result of better eating decisions.

You'll end up eating more advantageous foods like turmeric, which will add to your general feelings of well-being and health.

Hypnotherapy is somewhat similar to changing light. It requires almost no exertion, yet it can light up your life like you never thought conceivable.

If you need to lose weight for good, at that point, you ought to genuinely think about a hypnotic gastric band. Our unimaginable treatment can securely and, for all time, change your relationship with food. Inquisitive? Here are bits of primary data on hypnotic gastric bands.

1. Hypnosis is natural

The primary thing to recollect is that there is nothing to be frightened of with regards to hypnosis. Such a large number of legends and misguided judgments encompass it; however, hypnosis is really a usually happening state. Consider how relaxed you feel when you are fascinated in an extraordinary film or tuning in to a splendid bit of music. That is all that will transpire during a hypnotic gastric band session, and you will feel absolutely unconscious of the progression of time or your environmental factors.

2. More secure than surgery

An ever-increasing number of people are choosing weight loss surgery; however, this accompanies a great deal of vulnerabilities. Any activity conveys the danger of confusion, and regardless of whether that goes easily, you could wind up building up a disease a short time later. There is zero chance of any evil impacts with gastric band hypnotherapy. There is no recuperation time after your session, and you will have returned to typical and ready to carry on your everyday life immediately. Zero dangers, yet such a significant number of remunerations.

3. It's not simply hypnosis

Many individuals accept that hypnotic gastric band treatment uses, well, hypnosis. That couldn't possibly be more off-base, however. One of the generally secret realities about gastric band hypnotherapy is that it utilizes various strategies from different orders. Our sessions use parts of Cognitive Behavior Therapy (CBT), Time Perspective Therapy, NLP (Neuro-Linguistic Programming), Hypnosis, Guided Imagery, Mindfulness Techniques, and Pause Button Therapy to convey an extremely exhaustive treatment.

4. Changes how you eat

Hypnotic gastric band treatment is certifiably not a transient fix. It truly assists with getting to the base of any issues you have with food. Once those have been identified, you will have the option to change your relationship with eating for good. So as opposed to setting out on a massively restrictive accident diet which you can't keep up, you will have the option to move past any yearnings that you have for unhealthy foods, in the long run losing your desire for them inside and out.

5. Gives you certainty

Just as helping you to change truly, hypnosis for weight loss will likewise help you intellectually. It encourages you to relinquish negative convictions, which will make you feel considerably more certain about respect to your body. Having that recently discovered certainty will likewise fill you with the conviction that you can lose the weight that you have needed to for a considerable length of time, and you will have the option to accomplish your goals.

There is No Surgery

The Gastric Band Hypnosis strategy isn't careful, yet a sheltered option in contrast to surgery. Utilizing inventive forefront hypnotic innovation, a Virtual Gastric Band can be 'fitted,' giving you similar feelings that would be knowledgeable about surgery, however, without the uneasiness, time, burden, and cost. You will have the option to discharge weight consistently and securely. The impact is that you will start to eat a lot of little portions promptly and settle on more beneficial decisions. Engle Hypnotherapy causes you to understand the issue isn't with food, yet with your relationship with food.

Will It Work for Me?

It will work for you if you genuinely need it to and have a sensible creative mind. Close your eyes and envision a red entryway before you with a white ivory entryway handle. Would you be able to see it? If not, would you be able to envision that it's there? You need just permit yourself to deeply unwind with the goal of hypnotherapy to work for you. As the program proceeds, you will feel liberated in your mind and ease the burden from emotional weights.

In the trance state, you accomplish incredibly profound unwinding over an extended timeframe. The procedure will be a pleasure as opposed to weight. Your virtual gastric band results will influence your mind and your body. Every hypnosis session is custom-made to the specific and stated goals came to by the client and myself during the underlying assessment. The essential explanation this will work for you is that it is the main program that can wipe out your desires while simultaneously working with the emotional eating that caused the weight gain in any case. Taking care of the issue at the source is the best way to get lasting results.

Is Virtual Gastric Band Hypnosis Tailored to the Individual?

All together for the program to be successful, it must be custom fitted to your individual needs. Cutout sessions don't exist at Engle Hypnotherapy. Virtual gastric band hypnosis offers emotional mending just as your weight goal came to and effectively kept up.

Notwithstanding expelling food yearnings, we likewise dispense with negative emotional recollections; we don't dispose of the memory, obviously. However, we discharge any negative emotions you identified with the memory. The discharge is custom-made specifically to the client's one of a kind circumstance and viewpoint. The emotional part of weight gain is a major issue, and care must be taken to guarantee that when the weight is discharged, it is welcomed by a renewed individual, carrying on with another lifestyle, with a healthy emotional life.

Hypnotherapy isn't for everybody. It's just for those that are genuinely prepared to change how they feel about food. Those that don't need it to work will see almost no results.

Saying this doesn't imply that that being suspicious will hurt the procedure because it won't. Wariness is healthy, and those that come into it suspicious are consistently the ones that are most astounded when they understood that they had been mesmerized and their emotions have been mended.

CHAPTER SIX: HYPNOSIS PORTION CONTROL SESSION

Habits rule our lives and shape our present reality, yet it likewise shapes our future reality. Portion control is viewed as perhaps the main motivation why people gain weight, and although it may not sound useful to a few, it's really something that can represent the moment of truth in your weight loss journey.

During hypnotherapy, you need to be in control of your mind, which will permit you to control your habits and propensities you have easily. There are numerous reasons why people indulge. Some may not say that people settle on the choice to do as such, which implies it's likewise viewed as unmindful eating.

The most effective method to OVERCOME PORTION CONTROL AND OVEREATING DIFFICULTIES

We as a whole need food to endure, but when does the need food arrive at a point where it results in overeating and overindulging? When is it essential to take a look at yourself, make a stride back, and quit eating?

Each individual who has an unhealthy relationship with food sees it comparably. It frequently fills in as a method for solace and security that permits us to persuade ourselves that it is worthy of devouring food wildly and without intuition. Needless to state, unless you are prepared in nourishment or highly esteem thinking about your prosperity, you most likely don't have an exceptionally positive relationship with food.

CHANGE YOUR EATING HABITS

If you've perceived the need to construct a superior relationship with food, and you might want to find progressively about hypnosis for weight loss and to kick your bad habits, you need to identify the underlying reason adding to your concern. Since eating introduces itself as a type of impermanent pressure help and occupies us from feeling emotions like pressure, trouble, tension, and outrage, it's something we tend to incline toward at any rate eventually in our lives. Given that publicizing organizations are specialists at giving defective society foods that may appear to be engaging or are shrouded in to some degree "dietary-accommodating" content, we have embraced the conviction that it is alright to devour artificial food or whatever promoting recommends to us. We have similarly instructed ourselves that eating unhealthy food goes about as an award for whatever we're doing well.

Try not to PUNISH YOURSELF

For example, disclosing to yourself that you can eat

anything you desire throughout the end of the week after five weekdays of clean eating is totally off-base. We should not be feeling like we are rebuffing ourselves by eating a healthy, adjusted eating regimen. It should turn out to be natural to us as we receive a healthy lifestyle.

The initial step to successfully utilizing hypnosis for weight loss is identifying the reasons you battle to accomplish whatever it is you need. While experiencing self-hypnosis, you should figure out how to address your food fixation and transform it into something valuable, for example, inspiration to not feel as frail or wasteful as you do at your present weight or state of wellbeing.

Before you start with your session, you ought to recognize the motivation behind why your goal appears to be so far off, just as what it is that is keeping you away from accomplishing it.

WHAT WILL THE HYPNOTHERAPY SESSION BE LIKE?

During an expert hypnotherapy session, an advisor will, for the most part, ask you a rundown of inquiries identified with weight loss, including questions regarding your eating routine and exercise habits. Since you are directing the therapy session all alone, you can basically go over your day by day schedule and habits. Sometimes, it assists with recording both your positive and negative habits to see where you need to improve. You need to format the entirety of the data before you and spotlight what you need to improve during your session. Recording your goals will likewise help you develop a clearer image of where you'd prefer to go. Remember that self-hypnosis is entirely up to you, so you need to submit and remain restrained all through the 21 days.

This period is feasible for most people and sets a benchmark for yourself without making a dedication that is too enormous.

Since you need to reframe your food compulsion, it's critical to speak the truth about bad habits with yourself, which could incorporate anything from voraciously consuming food, emotional eating, overeating, or deceiving yourself to accept that you need more food or most usually blamed, disclosing to yourself that you'll begin an eating regimen on Monday.

Social occasion the important data about yourself and your habits will enable you to find what you need to address and spotlight on.

THE IMPORTANCE OF SETTING GOALS

Taking part in hypnotherapy, you will have the option to improve your certainty through positive proposals set out to cause you to feel enabled, reevaluate your inward voice, which will remind you to keep a positive and healthy mindset, imagine yourself accomplishing your weight loss goals, identify unconscious patterns that prompted your present unhealthy lifestyle, as dispose of any dread you may have in achieving your goals.

You most likely didn't realize that you could live in dread of accomplishing your goals. It sounds silly, but changing yourself or how you live could introduce itself as upsetting as well. Frequently people don't accomplish their goals because they are frightened of leaving their customary range of familiarity. Since we can't flourish or develop without being awkward in life, it's essential to defeat such apprehensions. Hypnosis will address your habit patterns and permit you to expel it from your psyche. It will allow you to grow new and economical ways of dealing with stress. For example, with Hypnosis, you can picture yourself reacting to upsetting cooperation or circumstance and pick how you might want to respond soundly. You will likewise envision yourself eating healthy during the session to help you settle on better decisions and structure lasting eating habits.

Picture SUCCESS

To the individuals who don't battle with portion and longing for control, think that it's easy to adhere to their standard method of eating. Contrasted with somebody who is urgent and eats dependent on their feelings, Hypnosis is most likely the best strategy for self-improvement. It works by controlling responses and propensities, which has clearly prompted your entanglements and unhealthy relationship with food. During the hypnosis session, you are prescribed to figure out how to dispatch your food longings and dispose of bad habits encompassing portion control.

This encourages you to picture yourself having a lot more profitable relationship with food, which will set you up for success.

With Hypnosis, it appears to be senseless to concentrate only on weight loss. There are such a significant number of different variables included that ascribes whatever causes weight gain that you can rectify. Losing weight and accomplishing any wellbeing related goal is a journey that will show you a way of carrying on with your best life.

Step by step instructions to EAT THE RIGHT AMOUNT OF FOOD

To regain legitimate portion control and eat the right measure of food at every meal, you need to concentrate on eating the right kinds of food. At that point, you will have to keep up a fair eating regimen. It's consistently useful to lead a little exploration before you start with Hypnosis, mainly if your goal is to figure out how to diminish your portion sizes and stick to it. Although you know the reasons why you should, and that eating an excessive amount of food adds to the pointless store of fat that gets put away in your body, many individuals, despite everything, indulge in any case. It's essential to remind yourself that you shouldn't be living to eat, yet rather eat to live. When you've built up this standard, you can control your portion sizes, and, at last, lose weight.

If you practice Hypnosis or are as of now following an eating regimen and you're not losing weight, at that point, you most likely need to assess your portion sizes. You additionally need to tune in to your body and realize whether the sort of food you're expending is serving your body well. Carrying excess weight could be a result of overeating at meals. Likewise, overeating as often as possible is equivalent to eating a bad eating regimen; it's bad for your general wellbeing or your weight loss journey.

Digestion

Legitimate portion control alone won't cause you to lose all the weight; however, it will give you more vitality, mainly because continually being full places strain on our real procedures to work more enthusiastically. This incorporates your digestion, which, if not working effectively, could make you clutch excess weight, totally end your weight loss results, and cause you to feel awkward. Having weak digestion and lack of processing could act as a genuine medical problem and incorporate problematic manifestations, such as unending weariness, weight gain, gloom, cerebral pains, clogging, and sugar longings.

The term "portion control" refers to eating a sufficient measure of food. The amount of what you expend, along with the sort thereof, is required if your goal is weight loss. Frequently, people drive themselves to complete the food on their plate out of amenability or because we can't perceive that we've had enough.

To control your portion sizes, you can have a go at doing the accompanying:

- Eat gradually and be increasingly cognizant about what you eat.
- Take a glass of water 15 minutes before you eat. This will fill your stomach and keep you from eating a lot at a time.
- Maintain a strategic distance from smorgasbords or eating 2-for-bargains at cafés.
- Substitute sweet beverages with natively constructed carbonated beverages (You'll need a Sodastream Jet or Fizzi for this)
- Take photographs of your meals and spare them in an envelope with the goal that you can return to and look at the size of your meals outwardly. This will likewise assist you with remaining on target and continue improving.

WHY HYPNOSIS WORKS FOR PORTION CONTROL

You can actualize the previously mentioned strategies for controlling your portion sizes at meals, yet you, despite everything, need to figure out how to defeat bad habits. Eating enthusiastically is nothing to be pleased with, and food must be considered as fuel. Improving the nature of your food regularly assists with portion control and can help you settle on the right choices. We should be genuine; nobody needs to eat a major plate of broccoli. Concentrating on how eating little versus huge amounts of food causes you to feel will likewise assist you with overcoming any psychological connection or need you may need to devour the right portions of food.

When you figure out how to beat your battles with portion control, you will arrive at a deeply relaxed state of mind and feel engaged, as you won't feel like you need to defeat your oblivious any longer. You will currently at long last be in control.

IT'S NOT ALL YOUR FAULT

Beating portion control is an enormous test, yet it isn't something that can't be accomplished. It is particularly difficult to accomplish in the public eye today. What used to be viewed as appropriate portion sizes has now doubled in the previous 50 years. Since there is another age of people, it has likewise been standardized, which has been one of the principal commitments to expanded instances of corpulence.

To fix any difficulty you may have identified with expending an excessive number of calories daily, regardless of whether it's overeating or eating void calories, you should take part in mindfulness. This is something that must be educated without anyone else. It's anything but an ability, but instead a demonstration of making a stride back and recognizing what you are doing, for example, what you are expending, including the amount thereof.

CHAPTER SEVEN: WHY HYPNOSIS WORKS FOR PORTION CONTROL

Portion control can assume a significant job in accomplishing your wellbeing and weight goals. You may, as of now, be eating quite a few foods and taking fitting activity.

Yet, if you, despite everything, end up carrying excess weight, it could be because you are just expending excessively. Portion control can have a significant effect.

Great portion control won't simply make you slimmer - it gives you more vitality. Eating the right sum will mean your body really needs to work less difficult to process pointless excess food.

Portion control is about the right measure of food

The amount is as significant as quality with regards to getting your eating regimen right and shedding excess fat. An overdose of something that is otherwise good indeed can be harmful when you need to lose weight. However, it can be hard to know how, when, and the amount to chop down so you can genuinely start to see some improvement in reaching your weight goals.

For what reason is it so challenging to practice portion control?

Habit runs our lives substantially more than we understand. We eat because it's time to eat (even though you had a nibble only thirty minutes prior). We indulge out of pleasantness, or not having any desire to 'squander' what is on our plate, or because we are so used to stuffing ourselves that we have overlooked how to perceive when we've had enough.

Some sound judgment things can assist you with controlling portion size:

- You can deliberately eat more gradually - this allows your stomach to enlist its totality in your cerebrum and switch off your craving.
- You can begin your meal with soup - a low-calorie soup can be fulfilling and permit you to feel content with a lot of a little portion for your fundamental course.
- You can utilize the old little plate trick - so you truly need to eat little portions.
- You can keep away from buffets and overlook 'uber meal' bargains.

Why hypnosis is an integral asset for

portion control

Incredible as the entirety of the above counsel seems to be, you, despite everything, need to conquer habit and impulse, which is the place hypnosis can truly help. Food is likened fuel, and fuel must be of the right quality and amount. Envision attempting to place more fuel into your vehicle when it's full. It simply doesn't bode well.

The Portion Control hypnosis session will bring you into a deeply relaxed state and rapidly train your unconscious mind to know naturally when to disregard excess food and permit your absorption to be a great deal more agreeable. You will rediscover the delight of being on top of what your own body actually needs for sustenance.

Some inexpensive food portions are two to five times huge than they were 50 years prior, adding to "portion twisting," a wonder where we have a flawed discernment and believe oversize portions to be ordinary.

For some uplifting news, certain practices may really make it simpler to control your portions. The following are tips and deceives to helping you deal with your portions while shedding a couple of pounds along the route without feeling at all pieces denied.

1. Keep the half-plate rule

Nobody got fat eating leafy foods. While a banana may

have a bigger number of calories than a cup of melon, getting a charge out of a banana won't make you fat. Likewise, while a cup of carrots contains a bigger number of calories than a cup of lettuce, this orange sweet-tasting veggie won't fill you out. Foods grown from the ground are stacked with fiber and water, helping you feel full while also giving your body nutrients, minerals, and cancer prevention agents useful for your wellbeing.

Size it up: Serve half of your plate with rich foods grown from the ground at every meal. Rehearsing portion control will feel a mess less difficult.

2. Blend and match

To practice portion-control viably, you would prefer not to feel hungry. To keep a strategic distance from such feelings, I propose eating foods that contain supplements that advance feelings of completion. Protein, fiber, and heart-healthy fats work. Along these lines at every meal, have a go at "blending and coordinating:" eating a mix of foods to keep you satisfied. Incorporate protein-rich foods, for example, fish, chicken, eggs, beans, and grass-took care of hamburger; fiber-rich organic products, vegetables, and entire grains (earthy colored rice, sweet potato, quinoa); and a sprinkling of healthy fats including olive oil, avocado, nuts, and seeds.

Size it up: A yummy- - and filling- - supper incorporates flame broiled salmon, cooked asparagus and cauliflower, and a cup of quinoa.

3. Smart size your dishes (and your spoons!)

The extensive examination has demonstrated that the size of our plates, bowls, and even utensils (truly, spoons!) can assume a significant job in the measure of food we eat. The bigger the plate, the more we serve ourselves and will, in general, eat.

Eating off of a bigger plate can really be a decent strategy for servings of mixed greens and veggies that we need to eat a greater amount of. Furthermore, not all portion-control strategies are tied in with eating less. In any case, for a pasta meal, I'd positively propose cutting back your bowl.

Spoon sizes and drinking glasses have any kind of effect as well!

Specialists announced that people drank more wine when their glass was greater. Bigger wine glass may change our impression of how much wine establishes a portion. It may drive us to drink quicker and arrange more.

Size it up: Want to appreciate a frozen yogurt treat in the long pooch stretches of summer? Utilize a little bowl and a teaspoon rather than a tablespoon.

4. Make a clench hand and utilize your hand as portion control

Your hand can probably be the best instrument around to assist you with checking portion sizes.

When you go out to eat, you're not liable to bring along a food scale and estimating cups; however, you generally have your hand.

Since such a large number of us exaggerate our starch portion (think rice, pasta, and potato), I encourage clients to make a clench hand and appreciate a healthy 1-cup portion as opposed to restricting starch inside and out.

This strategy isn't a precise science (all things considered, we as a whole have different size hands), yet it sure proves to be useful.

• a clench hand = 1 cup of rice, pasta, grain

• palm-space of your hand = 3 ounces of poultry or beef

• 2 fingers (a gesture of goodwill) = 2 ounces of cheddar

• twisted thumb joint = 1 tablespoon of oil or nutty spread

Size it up: Want to remember an incidental serving of red meat for your eating regimen, without trying too hard? Think a palm's worth. Also, add bunches of brilliant veggies to balance your plate.

5. Try not to venture out from home without your checkbook and dental floss

Picturing ordinary items can likewise be an incredible method to gauge serving sizes. Look at these recognizable things to help hold your portions in line. For extra visuals, look at my book The Portion Teller Plan.

• baseball = 1 cup of starch (rice, pasta, potatoes)

• deck of cards = 3-4 ounces of poultry or meat

• checkbook = 4 ounces white fish

• shot glass = 2 tablespoons oil or serving of mixed greens dressing

• bundle of dental floss = 1 ounce of a treat: a treat or bit of chocolate

Size it up: No need to restrict healthy grains from your supper plate. Fill half of your plate with your preferred veggies, a fourth of the plate healthy protein (1-2 decks of cards), and the other quarter (think one baseball's worth!) with a healthy grain, for example, wild rice, entire wheat pasta, or whole sorghum.

6. Enjoy, on occasion

It is OK to incorporate every day treat to shield you from feeling denied and to make your eating arrangement agreeable. This practice makes it simpler to practice portion-control and adhere to a healthy food plan as long as possible.

Size it up: Enjoy an incidental glass of wine with supper or a treat for dessert. Incorporate a huge bowl of blended berries as well!

7. Stock up on baggies and little compartments

An exhaustive report from scientists affirmed that bigger portions and bundles add to overeating. We will, in general, eat more when our food bundles are greater! What's more, we don't feel fuller.

Rather than encircle ourselves with allurement, I propose purchasing single-serving bundles or pre-portioning your preferred bites and placing them into baggies you can get when you are ravenous.

Size it up: Keep little holders helpful as well so you can store extras in immaculate portions.

8. Slow down, you move (and eat) excessively quick

Here's my lunch break. At the point when you are delayed down in all parts of your life, you will, in general, be increasingly mindful and are commonly more in line with your body's needs. You additionally wind up eating less! A successful victory!

Size it up: Savor your meal, make the most of your eating friend, and take in the middle of chomps.

CHAPTER EIGHT: HOW TO EAT THE RIGHT MEASURE OF FOOD

Odds are you've found out about the "healthy eating pyramid" sooner or later, and are entirely well across which foods you ought to and shouldn't eat for ideal wellbeing.

However, have you been trained what amount of food you should really be putting on your plate?

The absence of mindfulness about portion sizes is regularly the explanation people battle to control their weight.

Australia's official dietary rules suggest that people comprehend what it feels like to be "peckish" or "hungry," and use "completion" to check the amount to eat.

In any case, intuitive eating can be a test, which is why we need to investigate what's on our plates.

What should your plate resemble?

"We have grown up with the possibility that protein is the best and likewise to fill plates with bunches of pasta and rice."

"However, we need to rejig this by including more veggies and diminishing the size of the grain and carbohydrate-based foods, just as the proteins."

"Essentially, the reason is a fourth of the plate is loaded up with entire grains, things like pasta or bread or a bland vegetable like potatoes or sweet potato."

"Another quarter of the plate ought to be protein; a little bit of steak, a large portion of a cup of vegetables or two huge eggs, essentially something that fits in the palm of your hand."

At last, the last half should be a bright blend of veggies, like a plate of mixed greens or sautéed vegetables.

Getting portion sizes right

Lamentably, portion size can be dubious from the outset and may set aside some effort to get right.

In this way, when beginning, here are a few things to consider.

Check your plate size

Studies have discovered the physical size of a plate impacts the amount we eat.

Joel cautions plates have increased after some time, which can prompt overeating.

To battle this, utilize course sized dishes to hold your amounts under tight restraints.

Measure your food

It's not for everybody, except estimating portions will guarantee consistency.

Nutritionists state for "a most extreme effect," do your exploration to ensure you are getting the portions right.

It's tied in with taking a look at your calorie admission and the amount you need at that point modifying the proportion to suit.

Prep ahead: The straightforward intensity of meal arranging

A standard serve of:

Vegetable is about 75g (about ½ a cup of green or orange vegetables, ½ cup of cooked dried or canned beans or one cup of a plate of mixed greens).

Natural product is about 150g (around one banana or apple, two little kiwi organic products or apricots, or one cup of diced organic product).

Grain is about 400kJ (119 calories), for example, one cut of bread, ½ a roll, ½ a cup of cooked rice or pasta, or one crumpet.

Protein is 500-600kJ (119-143 calories), for example,

65g of lean red meat, 80g of lean poultry, 100g of cooked fish filet, two eggs, or 170g of tofu.

Dairy: 500-600kJ (119-143 calories), one cup of milk, 40g of hard cheddar, ½ cup of ricotta cheddar, or 200g of yogurt.

Serving versus Portion

The Dietary Guidelines depict three USDA Food Patterns, every one of which remembers slight varieties for sums suggested from different food gatherings. For example, people 50 or more established after the Healthy U.S.- Style Eating Pattern pick foods consistently from the accompanying:

- Vegetables — 2 to 3 cups
- Natural products — 1½ to 2 cups
- Grains — 5 to 8 ounces
- Dairy — 3 cups (without fat or low-fat)
- Protein foods — 5 to 6½ ounces
- Oils — 5 to 7 teaspoons

Does this mean you need to gauge or gauge everything you eat? Not so much. A few people discover it assists with estimating things cautiously from the start, yet once you become accustomed to your new eating arrangement, exact estimation likely won't be essential. Be that as it may, what precisely is a serving? Furthermore, is that different from a portion?

A "serving size" is a standard measure of food, for example, a cup or an ounce. Serving sizes can help you while picking foods and when looking at things while shopping, they are not proposals for the amount of a specific food to eat.

The term "portion" signifies the amount of food you are served or the amount you eat. A portion size can differ from meal to meal. For instance, at home, you may serve yourself two little hotcakes in a single portion; however, at a café, you may get an enormous heap of flapjacks as one portion. Portion size may likewise be greater than a serving size. For instance, the serving size on the Nutrition Facts name for your preferred grain might be 1 cup; however, you may present yourself with 1½ cups in a bowl.

Portion size can be difficult when eating out. To monitor your portion sizes, have a go at requesting a couple of little tidbits rather than a huge entrée. Or then again, you could share an entrée with a companion, or eat simply half and request a take-out holder for the rest. Put the extras in the cooler at the earliest opportunity. At that point, appreciate them the following day for lunch or supper.

TIP: SNACKING

Tidbits are alright, as long as they are keen on food decisions. If you need an evening jolt of energy or after-supper nibble, have a bit of organic product, or spread nutty spread or low-fat cream cheddar on whole wheat toast. Remember to remember snacks for your everyday food check. For example, 1 tablespoon of nutty spread on a cut of whole wheat toast checks toward the protein foods gathering and the gathering of the grain. A few thoughts for healthy eating include:

Have an ounce of cheddar with some entire grain wafers, a holder of low-fat or without fat yogurt, or a 1-ounce portion of unsalted nuts.

Put natural products rather than candy in the bowl on your end table.

Keep a compartment of washed, raw vegetables in the refrigerator along with hummus or other healthy plunges.

To restrict your portion's sizes, don't eat from the sack. Tally out a serving, and set the pack aside.

At the point when you are out and need a tidbit, don't be enticed by a pastry. Instead, bring a custom made path blend in a plastic pack when you go out. If you need to purchase a tidbit while you are in a hurry, get an apple or banana—most accommodation stores convey them.

CHAPTER NINE: HYPNOTIC LANGUAGE PATTERNS

Sometimes observed as dull and vile artistry, a mysterious force, or as something just heavyweight etymologists can get to grasps with, hypnotic language is, in reality, exceptionally clear. By definition, hypnotic language is intended to deliver a hypnotic trance. Since trance is basically a profoundly engaged state of consideration, the hypnotic language will be a language that concentrates and turns it inwards.

Have you heard somebody utilize hypnotic language patterns so breathtakingly that part of you just went, "Amazing! How on earth do you get the chance to be that acceptable!"?

Maybe it was only a solitary expression articulated by the trance inducer that totally flipped things around for the client, or perhaps it was a longer hypnotic enlistment that wove together a charming mix of story, cadence, and tone shift with a cunning cluster of embedded proposals. In any case, whatever it was, you were in wonder.

1. Circumstances and logical results

One thing will make something else occur. It's connecting two things together.

"Breathing in and out will make you feel progressively relaxed."

NOTE: The word because can prompt circumstances and logical results.

"Because you're breathing in and out, you can loosen up more deeply now."

2. Complex Equivalent

One thing implies something else.

"The way that you're perusing this book implies you're learning these patterns at a profound level."

3. Mind Reading

At the point when you state something you don't know is totally evident. Progressed admirably, it shows up as though you're guessing what someone might be thinking. We'll give you an example to demonstrate this point.

"I realize that you're anxious to gain proficiency with these language patterns."

4. Lost Performative

A worth judgment where you've lost the entertainer. You don't have a clue who's made the worth judgment. Ever have a gut response of: "Says who?" Good possibility you've run over a lost performative.

"Young men will be young men," versus, "My companion's mother said young men will be young men."

"Unwinding is beneficial for you," versus, "My yoga educator said unwinding is beneficial for you."

"Hypnosis is extraordinary for your mind," versus, "Igor said hypnosis is incredible for your mind."

"You can unwind deeply when you close your eyes," versus, "My advisor said you can unwind deeply when you close your eyes."

"I can't lose weight!" versus "My mother disclosed to me, I can't lose weight!"

5. Modal Operators

There are two modal operators: need and plausibility.

Need – words you can utilize are must, need, should, need to, and shouldn't.

"I need to win."

"You need to close your eyes to unwind deeply."

"You need to need to stop smoking for hypnosis to work."

"You need to ace these language patterns to turn out to be progressively persuasive."

Plausibility – words you can utilize are can, might, could, can't, and won't.

"You can't avoid going into a trance."

"You can permit yourself to drift deeper into a trance, right?"

"You may have the option to see a bright future in front of you."

"You can turn out to be increasingly powerful if you ace these language patterns."

6. Widespread Quantifier

Solid speculation that is, in every case, valid or never obvious. There's no center ground. Words to utilize are never, everybody, nobody, and consistently.

"I can do anything right!"

"I generally mess up!"

"Everybody can go into a trance!"

"Nobody can oppose unwinding deeply when the right conditions are met!"

7. Nominalization

An action word that doubles as a thing. It's an endeavor to transform a procedure into a thing. For example, unwinding is a nominalization. It's the way toward unwinding.

"You can appreciate this unwinding."

"You may see your downturn dissolving endlessly."

"You'll appreciate this solace topping off your body."

8. Unspecified Verb

An action word that isn't appropriately depicted. You don't tell people how.

"Close your eyes and unwind."

"You can close your eyes and unwind."

"You can get stunned at your positive changes."

9. Label Question

A label question assists with debilitating and mollify obstruction. These are usually utilized in deals.

"You need to ace language patterns, don't you?"

"You can envision utilizing label questions, right?"

"You're showing signs of improvement handle on language patterns, right?"

"You're going to wrap up this book, right?"

10. Absence of Referential Index

A statement that neglects to identify a part of the audience's understanding.

Example: "An individual can go into a trance."

11. Relative Deletion

This is a verbal cancellation of what one thing is being contrasted with. There is no specific reference to what or who is being erased.

"You'll appreciate drifting deeper into a trance." Which makes one wonder – deeper or more than what?

"This is a better course to move in life." Better than what bearing?

12. Pace Current Experience

This is essentially expressing what's going on as far as somebody can tell. NOTE: You're not thinking about what's going on. You're just referencing/saying what's verifiable.

How about we clarify this with an example

"You've been perusing this book. You've either perused the whole book so far, or you've skimmed it a piece, and you've recently found out about pacing statements; maybe you can envision utilizing pacing statements later on, can you not?"

If you investigate that again, you'll notice a pattern. There were three verifiable statements. It was then caught up with a statement of probability.

Pacing statements help to "oil the track." Which is simply one more method of saying they move the discussion down the easiest course of action. You're getting an oblivious yes with each verifiable statement. At the point when you line them up with a mind reader, it's effortlessly acknowledged as obvious.

Maybe you need another example.

13. Double Bind

A double bind is a dream of decision. At least two prospects lead to a similar result.

These are basic in a business circumstance.

"Would you like to pay with money or Mastercard?"

"Would you like to sign the paperwork around here or in my office?"

"Would you like to sit in the trance seat or the hypnosis seat?"

"Would you like to go into a trance rapidly or gradually?"

14. Embedded Commands

An embedded command is a verbal command that stands out in contrast to everything else to your oblivious. What's the reason? To seed a particular thought in your client's unconscious mind.

Here's the place a great many people get entangled. Utilizing one embedded command won't have as reliable as an impact as a progression of embedded commands.

It's all the more a pattern for your oblivious to follow. The more you insert commands, the more your client's oblivious will pay heed. It'll see these as a separate message.

That is a long-winded clarification.

"You'll have the option to go into a trance when your oblivious drifts off... I don't know how profound you will drift into the trance or even notification a shift in your breathing, and as you keep on tuning in to the sound of my voice, you can turn out to be increasingly relaxed".

Inevitably of hearing these orders, your oblivious would get on and give close consideration. It would begin to follow these recommendations.

When utilizing inserted orders, it can help by using a descending affectation.

15. Conversational Postulate

These are an order camouflaged as an inquiry. It is mentioning an activity while posing an inquiry. Unknowingly you answer yes. When you're noting indeed, you're as of now finishing the activity. Likewise, with inserted orders, a downward emphasis can make these significantly progressively amazing.

"Would you be able to open the entryway?"

"Would you be able to go into a daze now?"

"Do you have the opportunity?"

"Would you be able to get the telephone?"

"Would you be able to get the entryway?"

"Would you be able to envision the entirety of the potential outcomes?"

English is an entirely special language. It's experienced a lot of modifications, has sucked up a lot of sentence structure and jargon from numerous different languages, and is pretty much a Frankensteinian creation. For students of English as a second language, this means inconvenience.

For local or close local speakers, this opens up an entire universe of plausibility. In particular, we can utilize the structure of language, the structure of thought, and set up some exceptionally amazing hypnotic language designs.

Hypnotic Language For Fun

One way to utilize hypnotic language designs is to have some good times simply. The equivalent syntactic structure that makes jokes amusing can assist us with creating thoughts the fill in as mind bombs of disarray. Most jokes depend on equivocalness, for instance. Indeed:

Q: Which working in your town has the most stories?

A: The library!

Ahhhh ha! Get it? A story in the primary setting is intended to mean the floors of a structure. But at the same time, it's the sort of story that starts with "Once upon a time."

There are likewise a few ambiguities that can be utilized for turning their cerebrums around and around. One such equivocalness is the accentuation vagueness. This is the point at which you have two sentences that don't have anything to do with one another, yet the final expression of one sentence is the main expression of the following sentence. For instance:

A day or two, I saw this dessert truck stops always have the skankiest ladies; however, they're reasonable.

Another uncertainty is something called an extension vagueness. Where you have a sentence like Green roses and trees, it's not exactly sure whether the green goes with the two blossoms and trees, or simply the blossoms. The way to utilize this is concocted a degree equivocalness that will be deciphered one way, and afterward, drop in some data that will cause it to appear as though it's the other way. This is the methodology behind the acclaimed Groucho Marx joke:

The previous evening I shot an elephant in my nightwear. How he got in my nightwear, I'll never know.

Hypnotic Language For Direct Hypnosis

If you need to have a fabulous time at parties, spellbind your companions and make them talk nonsense, clacking like chickens or overlooking their names, there are a lot of ways to do that. In the motion pictures, the trance inducer just strolls up and says, "Rest!" and it works. In any case, that is the motion picture. It's somewhat trickier. In any case, it's still entirely simple. The first is a comprehension of pacing.

Hypnotic Pacing Statements

If you need to get people's minds feeling tricky, utilize a

lot of pacing statements. These are statements that must be valid. You are perusing this sentence. You are perusing this sentence. Sooner or later, before you read that last sentence, you ate something. Presently you can recollect the flavor of that food. As you recall that, and how it tasted, you may ponder when we are going to discuss some hypnosis.

Pace What They Are Doing

Composing this is difficult since I can't see you (that you are aware of...), and along these lines can't generally say much regarding what you are doing. Be that as it may, if you are watching somebody, there are huge amounts of things you can say about what they are really doing. At the point when you state pacing statements, ensure they coordinate the pace of their relaxing. Also, use bunches of pacing association words. Here are a few models that you may utilize if you were doing this for genuine at a gathering.

As you tune in to my voice...

What's more, take in...

Also, out...

You can sense the air in the room...

As it feels on your skin...

What's more, as you unwind back...

In that seat...

You can turn out to be considerably progressively agreeable...

What's more, consider how loosening up it is...

To simply tune in to my voice...

Also, become considerably progressively relaxed....

Elusive Slope Hypnotic Language

This is the point at which you begin to obscure the line between what they are truly doing and what you need them to do. In the long run, you need them to unwind totally, close their eyes, and comply with your voice totally. The more you loosen up the assortment of pacing statements and gradually blend them into leading statements, the more devoted they will be.

Interfacing Words

Um, huh?

There are many elusive words to interface what they are doing and what you need them to do. We will call what they are doing X, and what you need them to do Y.

As you X, you can perceive that it is so natural to Y...

The more you X, the simpler it is to Y...

Each time you X, you envision how great it feels good to Y...

Tuning in to my voice and X makes it so regular to Y...

At the point when They Are Deep In Trance

This is basically the structure of direct hypnosis. Watch them cautiously, utilize two or three pacing statements for each leading statement. At that point, the leading statement turns out to be valid and can be used for the following pacing statement. Utilize that pacing statement (which used to be a leading statement) along with another unadulterated pacing statement (something they are doing all alone) and give them another leading statement.

The longer you keep this up, the simpler it will be for them to keep obeying you. Prop up further and further until you make them fold their arms like a chicken or something.

Secret Hypnotic Language Patterns

Did You Really Just Say That?

The best hypnotic language design is the inserted order. An order is essentially a basic structure, a short statement like "turn left," or "include water." When utilized as an installed order, you basically put it in a sentence. For instance, think about the accompanying sentence:

A few days ago, I was tuning in to the radio, and the person said if you do situps consistently, you'll begin to feel better, and that will assist you with having a superior point of view.

It would appear that an ordinary statement, you'd get notifications from a typical individual is the way it's composed. In any case, think about the accompanying modifications:

A few days ago, I was tuning in to the radio, and the person said if you do sit-ups consistently, you'll begin to feel better, and that will assist you with having a superior point of view.

If you state the parts that are underlined marginally differently, the audience will see them as being orders, however, on an inner mind level. You state them like an order, where the final word is said with a marginally bring down volume than the rest. What's more, when you state the last word, you delay only a smidgen before proceeding.

CHAPTER TEN: BENEFITS OF EATING HEALTHY AND DETOXIFYING

A healthy diet includes an assortment of fruits and vegetables of numerous hues, entire grains and starches, high fats, and lean proteins.

Eating healthy additionally means staying away from foods with high measures of included salt and sugar.

Let's take a gander at the main advantages of a healthful diet, just as the proof behind them.

1. Weight loss

There are numerous advantages to eating healthfully.

Losing weight can assist with lessening the risk of interminable conditions. If an individual is overweight or hefty, they have a higher risk of building up a few conditions, including:

- heart disease
- non-insulin subordinate diabetes mellitus
- poor bone thickness
- a few diseases

Entire vegetables and fruits are lower in calories than most handled foods. An individual hoping to get in shape ought to lessen their calorie admission to close to what they require every day.

Determining a person's calorie prerequisites is simple, utilizing dietary rules distributed by the United States government.

Keeping up a healthy diet free from prepared foods can assist an individual with staying within their daily limit without tallying calories.

Fiber is one component of a healthy diet that is especially significant for overseeing weight. Plant-based foods contain a lot of dietary fiber, which assists with directing craving by causing people to feel fuller for longer.

In 2018, analysts found that a diet that is wealthy in fiber and lean proteins resulted in weight loss without the need to check calories.

2. Decreased malignant growth risk

An unhealthful diet can prompt weight, which may expand an individual's risk of creating malignancy. Weighing within a healthful range may lessen this risk.

Likewise, in 2014, the American Society of Clinical Oncology revealed that stoutness added to a more terrible viewpoint for people with the disease.

Notwithstanding, diets wealthy in fruits and vegetables may assist with ensuring against disease.

In a different report from 2014, scientists found that a diet that is wealthy in fruits decreased the risk of malignant growth in the upper gastrointestinal tract. They additionally found that a diet wealthy in vegetables, fruits, and fiber brought down the risk of colorectal disease and that a diet wealthy in fiber decreased the risk of malignant liver growth.

Numerous phytochemicals found in fruits, vegetables, nuts, and vegetables go about as cancer prevention agents, which shield cells from harm that can cause disease. Some of these cancer prevention agents include beta-carotene, lycopene, and vitamins A, C, and E.

Preliminaries in people have been uncertain; however, the results of the research center and creature contemplates have connected certain cell reinforcements to a decreased rate of free extreme harm related to malignant growth.

3. Diabetes management

Eating a healthy diet can assist an individual with diabetes to:

- get thinner, if required
- oversee blood glucose levels

- retain blood pressure and cholesterol within target ranges
- forestall or postpone confusions of diabetes

It is paramount for people with diabetes to constrain their admission of foods, including sugar and salt. It is likewise best to stay away from singed foods high in immersed and trans fats.

4. Heart health and stroke counteraction

As indicated by figures distributed in 2017, the same number as 92.1 million people in the U.S. have, at any rate, one kind of cardiovascular disease. These conditions principally include the heart or blood vessels.

As shown by the Heart and Stroke Foundation of Canada, up to 80 percent of instances of untimely heart disease and stroke can be forestalled by making lifestyle changes, for example, expanding levels of physical activity and eating healthfully.

There are some proofs that vitamin E may forestall blood clumps, which can prompt heart assaults. The accompanying foods contain significant levels of vitamin E:

- almonds
- peanuts
- hazelnuts

- sunflower seeds
- green vegetables

The clinical network has long perceived the connection between trans fats and heart-related illnesses, for example, coronary heart disease.

If an individual kills trans fats from the diet, this will diminish their degrees of low-thickness lipoprotein cholesterol. This kind of cholesterol makes plaque gather within the veins, expanding the risk of heart assault and stroke.

Diminishing blood pressure can likewise be fundamental for heart health, and restricting salt admission to 1,500 milligrams a day can help.

Salt is added to many handled and fast foods, and individuals who want to bring down their blood pressure should maintain a strategic distance from these.

5. The health of the people to come

Youngsters take in most health-related practices from the grown-ups around them, and guardians who model healthful eating and exercise habits will, in general, pass these on.

Eating at home may likewise help. In 2018, scientists found that youngsters who regularly had meals with their families ate a greater number of vegetables and less sugary foods than their friends who ate at homeless habitually.

Also, kids who take an interest in planting and cooking at home might be bound to settle on healthy dietary and lifestyle choices.

6. Solid bones and teeth

Kids take in healthful practices from their folks.

A diet with sufficient calcium and magnesium is important for solid bones and teeth. Keeping the bones healthy is imperative in forestalling osteoporosis and osteoarthritis further down the road.

The accompanying foods are wealthy in calcium:

- low-fat dairy products
- broccoli
- cauliflower
- cabbage
- canned fish with bones
- tofu
- vegetables

Likewise, numerous oats and plant-based milk are fortified with calcium.

Magnesium is copious in many foods, and the best sources are verdant green vegetables, nuts, seeds, and entire grains.

7. Better mind-set

Developing proof proposes an intimate connection between diet and disposition.

In 2016, specialists found that a diet with a high glycemic burden may cause expanded side effects of sorrow and fatigue.

A diet with a high glycemic load incorporates many refined carbohydrates, such as those found in soda, cakes, white bread, and rolls. Vegetables, entire fruit, and whole grains have a lower glycemic load.

While a healthful diet may improve general temperament, it is fundamental for people with melancholy to look for clinical consideration.

8. Improved memory

A healthy diet may help forestall dementia and subjective decay.

An investigation from 2015 identified supplements and foods that ensure against these antagonistic impacts. They saw the accompanying as valuable:

- nutrient D, C, and E
- omega-3 fatty acids
- flavonoids and polyphenols
- fish

Among different diets, the Mediterranean diet joins a large number of these supplements.

9. Improved gut health

The colon is brimming with normally happening microscopic organisms, which assume significant jobs in digestion and assimilation.

Certain strains of microorganisms additionally produce nutrients K and B, which advantage the colon. These strains likewise help to battle unsafe microscopic organisms and infections.

A diet low in fiber and high in sugar and fat changes the gut microbiome, expanding irritation in the territory.

In any case, a diet wealthy in vegetables, fruits, vegetables, and entire grains gives a blend of prebiotics and probiotics that help great microorganisms to flourish in the colon.

Aged foods, like yogurt, kimchi, sauerkraut, miso, and kefir, are wealthy in probiotics.

Fiber is an effectively available prebiotic, and it is bottomless in vegetables, grains, fruits, and vegetables.

Fiber likewise advances regular solid discharges, which can assist with forestalling entrail malignant growth and diverticulitis.

10. Getting a decent night's rest

An assortment of elements, including rest apnea, can upset rest designs.

Rest apnea happens when the airways are over and again obstructed during rest. Risk factors include stoutness, drinking liquor, and eating an unhealthful diet.

Lessening the utilization of liquor and caffeine can help guarantee relaxing rest, regardless of whether an individual has rest apnea.

Brisk tips for a healthful diet

Trading soda pops for homegrown teas is a constructive change in an individual's diet.

There are a lot of little positive ways to improve the diet, including:

- trading soda pops for water and natural tea
- eating no meat for at any rate one day, seven days
- guaranteeing that produce makes up around 50 percent of every meal
- trading dairy animals' milk for plant-based milk
- eating entire fruits as opposed to drinking juices, which contain less fiber and frequently include included sugar

- staying away from handled meats, which are high in salt and may expand the risk of malignant colon growth
- eating increasingly lean protein, which can be found in eggs, tofu, fish, and nuts.

An individual may likewise profit by taking a cooking class and figuring out how to join more vegetables into meals.

Advantages OF DETOXIFYING

There is, by all accounts, an equivalent measure of alerts and proposals for detoxing, which can make it mistaking for the eventual detox dieter. For whatever length of time you utilize the presence of mind, adjust the detox diet to your own goals, and remain committed; there can be numerous advantages to detoxification.

I've sketched out a portion of the advantages you can expect by following a decent detox program:

1. Lifts your energy

By flushing the toxins out from your body, detoxification leaves you feeling progressively vigorous and enthusiastic. While you detox, you also stop the deluge of sugar, caffeine, trans fat, and saturated fat, and replace them with common foods, for example, fruits and vegetables. You get a characteristic energy help, one that comes without a resultant accident.

It's imperative to remain very much hydrated while on any detox program. This can likewise be a wellspring of expanded energy if you usually don't get enough water for the day.

2. Frees the body of any excess waste

The fundamental reason for detoxing is to permit your body to dispose of any excess waste it's been putting away. Detox programs are planned for animating the body to cleanse itself, including the liver, kidneys, and colons. Most present-day diseases are brought about by putting away waste in the body, which is why detoxifying is significant.

For instance, purifying the colon is a significant piece of the detoxing procedure because poisons need to leave the body, and an upheld up colon can make them be reintroduced into the body, as opposed to leaving as arranged. Considerably after the detox program, it is prescribed to proceed with a diet wealthy in dissolvable fibers to keep your body healthy.

3. Assists with weight loss

An analysis of detox diets is that they just assist you with losing weight for the time being. It helps, instead, if you see detox programs as a way to set up long-term eating habits and free yourself of unhealthy habits. Everything relies upon what you center around.

If you just consider the extreme decrease in calories and fast weight loss, you are bound to gain all that weight back when you stop. These provisional results won't last if you don't make it a point to supplant terrible foods with good ones and utilize your recently discovered energy to practice more and be increasingly dynamic in general.

4. More grounded immune system

Detoxifying your body likewise fortifies your immune system. Your organs are perfect and free to work as they should. Your body can curtail supplements better, including Vitamin C.

Great detox programs have a suggested admission of herbs, which help the lymphatic system. This system is a significant player in keeping you healthy long term. Many detox programs likewise center around light activities, which help to circle lymph liquid through the body and cause it to deplete, fortifying your immune system simultaneously.

5. Improved skin

Your skin is your biggest organ. Since detox programs improve your general health, it bodes well that your skin benefits the most.

Detox programs prescribe setting off to a sauna to take a sauna to enable the body to work out extra poisons. Numerous people are agreeably amazed by more precise, smoother skin toward the finish of their detox plan. It's additionally been accounted for that detoxing can help with skin inflammation, although the condition may compound before it shows signs of improvement as the poisons are discharged. You may find that your skin tingles or gets sketchy before clearing up, yet this is a piece of the procedure and is an indication that you're in good shape with your program. Persistence and devotion to the detox program is the thing that has a significant effect on progress and disappointment.

6. Better breath

A few people observe better common breath a long time into their detox program. One purpose behind terrible breath is a supported up colon. During a detox, you can get it out and get your stomach related system working great again. As a result, your breath will see a characteristic improvement over the coming weeks.

7. Administers healthy changes

Detox can be a month and a half or thereabouts, yet the changes it makes in your lifestyle are long term. A detox program can be your gateway to a healthier life.

You can use a detox program to help you execute those desires if you have addictions to sugar, caffeine, or seared or crunchy foods. If you purge the body and supplant those foods with healthier choices, you can retrain yourself and be bound to adhere to your new habits.

8. More clear reasoning

A purify benefits your body; however, it additionally

reinforces the state of your mind. Reflection is an extraordinary way to loosen up your mind and lower your feelings of anxiety.

While the detox is cleansing your body and purifying it of poisons, remember to concentrate on your emotional well-being simultaneously.

Detox adherents frequently state that they lose that feeling of fogginess and can think more plainly during a detox than when not on it. It bodes well, since a large number of the sugar-filled and fat-filled foods that encompass us every day will make us feel torpid and can factor intensely in the nature of our reasoning.

9. Healthier hair

A ton of herbs, nutrients, and minerals you devour during a detox directly affect making your hair healthier. At the point when your hair is healthy, it looks better and is harder to break. This is the reason it's essential to keep your body working at its maximum capacity through a regular detoxing methodology.

When your hair can become uninhibited by inner poisons, you'll see and feel the difference in your hair. In numerous occurrences, hair gets shinier, more grounded, and feels milder to the touch. What's more, numerous people on a detox program report that it recouped their hair loss because of male example sparseness.

10. Lighter feeling

Unrestricted by sugar and fat that make it lazy, your body will feel "lighter" as you progress through your detox diet.

There are a few reasons this would be the situation, particularly if you'll be doing a colon purification as a significant aspect of the program. When you quit eating foods that burden you and replace them with new natural fruits and vegetables, a lighter feeling will undoubtedly happen. Your body normally recharges the energy you lose for the duration of the day with the assistance of a decent, natural diet.

11. Hostile to maturing benefits

As of now, referenced, detoxing has long-term impacts, one of which is hostile to maturing.

One contributing element to the maturing procedure is the steady blast of poisons that our bodies need to fight each day. The trans-fats, sugar, and caffeine we feed our bodies every day remain in our systems for a long time, presenting free radicals and terrible poisons. Detoxing gives momentary advantages; however, those following the programs see long term benefits that battle untimely maturing. Be that as it may, for this to work, it is critical to change your lifestyle much after the detox program is done.

Adhering to an improved diet and getting day by day activity are incredible ways to ensure that you feel great every moment of your life.

12. Improved feeling of prosperity

An effective detox takes difficult work, devotion, and inspirational demeanor. Detoxing can be an incredible way to present a change in your lifestyle to improve things. At the point when you detox, you feel great, and when you feel great, beneficial things occur.

Whatever your purpose behind beginning a detox diet, regardless of whether it is losing weight or bringing down pressure, it is critical to keep the positive changes long after the detox program is finished.

At the point when you set up for prosperity, you will improve all aspects of your life. Merely this one change can help you build better connections, be progressively productive at work or in your diversions, and appreciate life to its maximum capacity.

CHAPTER ELEVEN: EATING HEALTHY EATING LESS UNHEALTHY

Everybody needs to have a healthy body that works well, and one of the essential keys to accomplishing ideal health is healthy eating. Notwithstanding, eating right can be a test, particularly when such a large number of foods are intensely handled or have included unhealthy fixings. Another enormous issue is the way advertisers make products sound healthier than they really are and attempt to make people content with eating less unhealthy, rather than really eating healthy.

Today there are numerous foods, especially with regards to bundled products, that are promoted to be healthier renditions of different foods. It is better to eat the healthier of two products; however, a considerable lot of these supposed "healthier" products don't really make you any healthier or even assist you with losing weight. These products are normally intended to cause people to feel better about eating foods that are as yet unhealthy, while not being the unhealthiest choice accessible.

For example, consider potato chips. Quite a while back, there were generally hardly any choices when it came to potato chips, with virtually every one of them being high in fat, and the principal differences between brands were things like shape and thickness. At that point, as people turned out to be more health-conscious, the offer of regular chips began declining, and organizations had to start making different kinds of chips to speak to more health-conscious purchasers.

As a result, numerous organizations came out with lower fat renditions of their chips, and lately, they began evacuating the unhealthiest types of fat (in part hydrogenated oils and trans-fats) chips. Different organizations began making prepared chips rather than singed chips, so the chips would contain less fat and be less unhealthy. Be that as it may, these changes were exceptionally simply made to get people to continue purchasing chips. By giving a healthier option in contrast to regular chips, it permits people to feel better or justify their choice to purchase chips.

It's just as picking a less unhealthy alternative in one way, or another makes it worthy, and the less unhealthy decision winds up being thought of as a healthy decision. While the healthier choice might be an improvement, it is typically only a minor improvement, and the "healthier" food is still a long way from healthy. Lower fat chips are as yet a significant wellspring of void calories, they do practically nothing to improve your health, and they will make you gain fat nearly as fast and effectively as regular chips.

A few people even gain more weight when they change from unhealthier food to a hardly healthier one because they feel like they can eat a greater amount of healthier food. Yet, they simply wind up eating increasingly all out calories, which prompts weight and fat gain. This can undoubtedly occur with products like the famous 100 calorie nibble pack foods.

These products are essentially lousy nourishment bundled in 100 calorie servings, and they are healthfully the same as the products found in bigger sacks. Notwithstanding, since they are showcased as having just 100 calories for every pack, people get the feeling that they are somehow or another better than regular sacks or boxed lousy nourishment. One hundred calorie packs are possibly better if they genuinely assist people with controlling their portion sizes. Yet, as a rule, people wind up eating various bundles or are left unsatisfied and wind up, discovering something else to eat. These kinds of products are unquestionable, more a contrivance than anything.

Rather than purchasing healthier renditions of unhealthy foods or bundles of unhealthy foods that are in littler servings, the perfect technique is basically to buy foods that are really healthy, not simply less unhealthy than regular low quality nourishments. Obviously, changing from extremely unhealthy food to a less unhealthy one might be an improvement, yet all things considered, it's anything but a change that will help you arrive at your health and wellness goals.

If you eat plenty of unhealthy foods, changing to less unhealthy variants of those foods is a decent spot to begin, yet don't let yourself become content with merely settling on those little changes in food choices. If you are genuinely genuine about improving your health and sustenance, at that point, your goal needs to include eating healthy foods as frequently as could be expected under the circumstances and not agreeing to eat foods that are just less unhealthy. At last, less unhealthy foods wind up being sufficiently bad, so don't stress a lot over correlations among foods and go for the foods you know are healthy.

Think, excluding natural products, when was the last time you saw showcasing to advance a healthier variant of broccoli, apples, or other normal produce? These foods are healthy, so there is no pressure to improve the renditions of these products. A healthier form of unhealthy food generally means it isn't precisely as terrible and all things considered, if food needs a healthier rendition, at that point, it is likely something you would prefer not to eat a whole lot in any case. Stick to common healthy foods, and you will improve your health and sustenance significantly more than if your goal is to eat less unhealthy foods.

Healthy versus Unhealthy Diets

In any event, 2.7 million people far and wide bite the dust every year as a result of not getting enough fruits and vegetables in their diets, as per the World Health

Organization. Eating healthy food rather than an unhealthy diet can assist you with getting all the fundamental supplements you need and cut off your risk for various health conditions.

Healthy diets are made up essentially of supplement rich foods, for example, vegetables, fruits and vegetables, entire grains, low-fat dairy products, lean protein and nuts, and seeds. Unhealthy diets are high in fat, soaked fat, trans fat, sodium, and included sugars. These diets frequently contain a ton of handled or quick foods that are high in calories; however, they don't contain numerous supplements. People following a healthy diet watch their portion sizes, so they keep up a healthy weight since both the amount and the nature of the food you eat is significant for a healthy diet.

Supplement Intake

If you eat healthy, you are bound to get enough of the supplements, like fiber, calcium, nutrient D, and potassium, which many Americans don't expend in adequate sums. Entire grains, vegetables, vegetables, fruits, and nuts give fiber; low-fat journal products and verdant green vegetables give calcium; fruits and vegetables like bananas, apricots, strawberries, avocado, and cucumber are acceptable wellsprings of potassium; and fish, eggs and fortified milk and squeezed orange contain nutrient D.

Disease Risk

Up to 40 percent of malignancies might be expected, to a limited extent, to following an unhealthy diet, unhealthy diets likewise increment your risk for Type 2 diabetes, heftiness, and heart disease. The World Health Organization assesses that around 2.6 million passings every year are because of stoutness related illnesses.

Contemplations

Preparing time and permitting yourself a little portion of a not precisely healthy treat now and again can assist you with adhering to a healthy diet. Following a healthy diet isn't the main thing that issues - you likewise need to make healthy lifestyle changes to limit your disease risk. Exercise regularly quit smoking and drink just with some restraint, if by any means.

CHAPTER TWELVE: FREE GUIDE FOR EATING HEALTHY

What is a healthy diet?

Eating a healthy diet isn't about exacting constraints, ridiculously meager, or denying yourself the foods you love. Or maybe it's tied in with feeling incredible, having more energy, improving your health, and boosting your state of mind.

Healthy eating doesn't need to be excessively convoluted. If you feel overpowered by all the clashing nourishment and diet exhortation out there, you're not the only one. It appears that for each master who reveals to you a specific food is beneficial for you, you'll discover another colloquialism, precisely the inverse. In all actuality, while some specific foods or supplements have been appeared to affect temperament beneficially, it's your general dietary example that is generally significant. The foundation of a healthy diet ought to be to supplant handled food with genuine food at whatever point conceivable. Eating food that is as close as conceivable to the way nature caused it to can have a tremendous effect on the way you think, look, and feel.

The essentials of healthy eating

While some extreme diets may recommend else, we as a whole need equalization of protein, fat, carbohydrates, fiber, nutrients, and minerals in our diets to continue a healthy body. You don't need to take out specific classes of food from your diet, yet select the healthiest alternatives from every classification.

Protein gives you the energy to get moving—and continue onward—while additionally supporting disposition and subjective capacity. A lot of protein can be hurtful to people with kidney disease; however, the most recent exploration proposes that a significant number of us need the most excellent protein, particularly as we age. That doesn't mean you need to eat creature products increasingly—an assortment of plant-based wellsprings of protein every day can guarantee your body gets all the basic protein it needs.

Fat. Not all fat is the equivalent. While terrible fats can wreck your diet and increment your risk of specific diseases, high fats ensure your mind and heart. Healthy fats, for example, omega-3s—are indispensable to your physical and passionate health. Remembering increasingly healthy fat for your diet can help improve your temperament, support your prosperity, and even trim your waistline.

Fiber. Eating foods high in dietary fiber (grains, fruit, vegetables, nuts, and beans) can help you remain regular and lower your risk for heart disease, stroke, and diabetes. It can likewise improve your skin and even assist you in getting more fit.

Calcium. Just as leading to osteoporosis, not getting enough calcium in your diet can likewise add to uneasiness, sorrow, and rest difficulties. Whatever your age or sexual orientation, it's fundamental to include calcium-rich foods in your diet, limit those that exhaust calcium, and get enough magnesium and nutrients D and K to assist calcium with carrying out its responsibility.

Carbohydrates are one of your body's principle wellsprings of energy. In any case, most should originate from mind-boggling, unrefined carbs (vegetables, entire grains, fruit) as opposed to sugars and refined carbs. Curtailing white bread, baked goods, starches, and sugar can forestall quick spikes in blood sugar, vacillations in the mind and energy, and development of fat, particularly around your waistline.

Doing the change to a healthy diet

Changing to a healthy diet doesn't need to be a win big or bust suggestion. You don't need to be great, you don't need to totally dispose of foods you appreciate, and you don't need to change everything at the same time—that typically just prompts cheating or abandoning your new eating arrangement.

A superior methodology is to make a couple of little changes, one after another. Keeping your goals humble can help you accomplish more in the long term without feeling denied or overpowered by a significant diet update. Consider arranging a healthy diet as various little, reasonable advances—like adding a plate of mixed greens to your diet once per day. As your small changes become a habit, you can keep on including increasingly healthy choices.

Setting yourself up for progress

To set yourself up for progress, attempt to keep things straightforward. Eating a healthier diet doesn't need to be confused. Rather than being excessively worried about tallying calories, for instance, think about your diet in terms of shading, assortment, and newness. Concentrate on dodging bundled and handled foods and deciding on increasingly new fixings at whatever point conceivable.

Plan your very own greater amount of meals. Preparing more meals at home can assist you with assuming responsibility for what you're eating and better screen precisely what goes into your food. You'll eat fewer calories and evade the synthetic added substances, including sugar and unhealthy fats of bundled and takeout foods that can leave you feeling tired, enlarged, and crabby, and intensify side effects of misery, stress, and nervousness.

Make the right changes. When decreasing unhealthy foods in your diet, it's imperative to supplant them with healthy other options. Replacing perilous trans fats with healthy fats (for example, exchanging singed chicken for flame-broiled salmon) will have a constructive outcome to your health. Swapping creature fats for refined carbohydrates, however, (for example, exchanging your morning meal bacon for a doughnut), won't bring down your risk for heart disease or improve your state of mind.

Peruse the names. It's imperative to know about what's in your food as producers frequently conceal a lot of sugar or unhealthy fats in bundled food, even food professing to be healthy.

Concentrate on how you feel in the wake of eating. This will help encourage healthy new habits and tastes. The healthier the food you eat, the better you'll feel after a meal. The more low-quality nourishment you eat, the almost sure you are to feel awkward, sick, or depleted of energy.

Drink a lot of water. Water helps flush our systems of waste products and poisons, yet a considerable lot of us experience life got dried out—causing sleepiness, low energy, and cerebral pains. It's not unexpected to confuse thirst with hunger, so remaining all-around hydrated will likewise assist you with settling on healthier food choices.

The way to a healthy diet is to eat the right measure of calories for how dynamic you are, so you balance the energy you devour with the energy you use.

If you eat or drink more than your body needs, you'll put on weight because the energy you don't utilize is put away as fat. If you eat and drink close to nothing, you'll get thinner.

You ought to likewise eat a broad scope of foods to ensure you're getting a decent diet, and your body is accepting all the supplements it needs.

It's suggested that men have around 2,500 calories per day (10,500 kilojoules). Ladies ought to have around 2,000 calories per day (8,400 kilojoules).

1. Base your meals on higher fiber dull carbohydrates

Dull carbohydrates should make up a little more than 33% of the food you eat. They include potatoes, bread, rice, pasta, and grains.

Pick higher fiber or wholegrain assortments, for example, wholewheat pasta, earthy colored rice, or potatoes with their skins on.

They contain more fiber than white or refined boring carbohydrates and can help you feel full longer.

Attempt to include at any rate one bland food with every principle meal. A few people think boring foods are fattening, but gram for gram, the starch they contain gives less than a large portion of the calories of fat.

Watch out for the fats you include when you're cooking or serving these sorts of foods because that is the thing that builds the calorie content – for instance, oil on chips, spread on bread, and creamy sauces on pasta.

2. Eat heaps of fruit and veg

It's suggested that you eat in any event five portions of an assortment of fruit and veg consistently. They can be new, solidified, canned, dried, or juiced.

Getting your 5 A Day is simpler than it sounds. Why not cleave a banana over your morning meal grain, or trade your standard early in the day nibble for a bit of new fruit?

A portion of new, canned, or solidified fruit and vegetables is 80g. A portion of dried fruit (which ought to be kept to mealtimes) is 30g.

A 150ml glass of fruit juice, vegetable juice, or smoothie additionally considers one portion, yet limit the sum you have to close to 1 glass a day as these drinks are sugary and can harm your teeth.

3. Eat more fish, including a portion of oily fish

Fish is a decent wellspring of protein and contains numerous nutrients and minerals.

Mean to eat in any event two portions of fish seven days, including in any event one portion of oily fish.

Oily fish are high in omega-3 fats, which may help forestall heart disease.

Oily fish include:

- salmon
- trout
- herring
- sardines
- pilchards
- mackerel
- Non-oily fish include:
- haddock
- plaice
- coley
- cod
- fish
- skate
- hake

You can browse new, solidified, and canned, yet recollect that canned and smoked fish can be high in salt.

Many people ought to eat more fish; however, there are suggested limits for certain kinds of fish.

Discover progressively about fish and shellfish.

4. Cut down on immersed fat and sugar

You need some fat in your diet; however, it's critical to focus on the sum and kind of fat you're eating.

There are two primary kinds of fat: soaked and unsaturated. An excess of immersed fat can expand the cholesterol measure in the blood, which builds the risk of creating heart disease.

By and large, men ought to have close to 30g of saturated fat a day. Ladies ought to have close to 20g of saturated fat a day.

Youngsters younger than 11 should have less saturated fat than grown-ups, yet a low-fat diet isn't reasonable for kids under 5.

Immersed fat is found in numerous foods, for example,

- fatty cuts of meat
- hotdogs
- spread
- hard cheddar
- cream
- cakes
- scones
- fat
- pies

Attempt to eliminate your soaked fat admission and

pick foods that contain unsaturated fats instead, for example, vegetable oils and spreads, oily fish, and avocados.

For a healthier decision, utilize a limited quantity of vegetable or olive oil, or decreased fat spread rather than margarine, fat, or ghee.

At the point when you have meat, pick lean cuts, and remove any noticeable fat.

A wide range of fat are high in energy, so they should just be eaten in modest quantities.

SUGAR

Regularly devouring foods and drinks high in sugar builds your risk of heftiness and tooth decay.

Sugary foods and drinks are frequently high in energy (estimated in kilojoules or calories), and if expended repeatedly, they can add to weight gain. They can likewise cause tooth decay, mainly if eaten between meals.

Free sugars are any sugars added to foods or drinks or discovered normally in nectar, syrups, and unsweetened fruit juices and smoothies.

This is the kind of sugar you ought to be eliminated, instead of the sugar found in fruit and milk.

Many bundled foods and drinks contain shockingly high

measures of free sugars.

Free sugars are found in numerous foods, for example,

- sugary, bubbly drinks
- sugary breakfast grains
- cakes
- scones
- baked goods and puddings
- desserts and chocolate
- mixed drinks

Food names can help. Use them to check how much sugar foods contain.

More than 22.5g of absolute sugars per 100g means the food is high in sugar, while 5g of complete sugars or less per 100g means the food is low in sugar.

Get tips on eliminating sugar in your diet

5. Eat less salt: close to 6g per day for grown-ups

Eating an excessive amount of salt can raise your blood pressure. People with hypertension are bound to create heart disease or have a stroke.

Regardless of whether you don't add salt to your food, you may, at present, be overeating.

Around seventy-five percent of the salt you eat is as of now in the food when you get it, for example, breakfast grains, soups, loaves of bread, and sauces.

Use food marks to assist you with chopping down. More than 1.5g of salt per 100g means the food is high in salt.

Grown-ups and youngsters matured 11 and over ought to eat close to 6g of salt (about a teaspoonful) a day. More youthful kids ought to have even less.

Get tips on eliminating salt in your diet

6. Get dynamic and be a healthy weight

Just as eating healthily, regular exercise may reduce your risk of quitting any funny business health conditions. It's additionally significant for your general health and prosperity.

Peruse increasingly about the advantages of activity and physical activity rules for grown-ups.

Being overweight or fat can prompt health conditions, such as type 2 diabetes, certain malignant growths, heart disease, and stroke. Being underweight could likewise influence your health.

Most grown-ups need to get in shape by eating fewer calories.

If you're attempting to get in shape, intend to eat less, and be progressively dynamic. Eating a healthy, adjusted diet can assist you in keeping up a healthy weight.

Check whether you're a healthy weight by utilizing the BMI healthy weight mini-computer.

Start the NHS weight loss plan, a 12-week weight loss direct that joins counsel on healthier eating and physical activity.

If you're underweight, see underweight grown-ups. If you're stressed over your weight, approach your GP or a dietitian for exhortation.

7. Try not to get parched

You need to drink a lot of liquids to stop you from getting dried out. The legislature prescribes drinking 6 to 8 glasses each day. This is notwithstanding the liquid you get from the food you eat.

All non-mixed drinks tally, however water, lower-fat milk, and lower-sugar drinks, including tea and espresso, are healthier choices.

Attempt to maintain a strategic distance from sugary delicate, and bubbly drinks, as they're high in calories. They're additionally awful for your teeth.

Indeed, even unsweetened fruit juice and smoothies are high in free sugar.

Your joined aggregate of drinks from fruit juice,

vegetable juice, and smoothies should not be more than 150ml per day, which is a little glass.

Make sure to drink more liquids during sweltering climate or while working out.

8. Try not to skip breakfast

A few people skip breakfast because they think it'll assist them with losing weight.

Be that as it may, a healthy breakfast high in fiber and low in fat, sugar, and salt can shape some portions of a decent diet and help you get the supplements you need for good health.

A wholegrain lower sugar grain with semi-skimmed milk and fruit cut over the top is a delectable and healthier breakfast.

Control: imperative to any healthy diet

What is the balance? Generally, it means eating just as much food as your body needs. You should feel fulfilled toward the finish of a meal, however not stuffed. For a considerable lot of us, the control means eating short of what we do now. Be that as it may, it doesn't mean killing the foods you love. Eating bacon for breakfast once every week, for instance, could be viewed as balance if you tail it with a healthy lunch and supper— yet not if you tail it with a crate of doughnuts and a hotdog pizza.

Do whatever it takes not to think about specific foods as "forbidden." When you boycott certain foods, it's reasonable to need those foods more, and afterward, feel like a disappointment if you surrender to enticement. Start by lessening portion sizes of unhealthy foods and not eating them as frequently. As you lessen your admission to unhealthy foods, you may end up longing for them less or considering them just incidental guilty pleasures.

Think little portions. Serving sizes have expanded as of late. When feasting out, pick a starter rather than a course, split a dish with a companion, and don't structure supersized anything. At home, visible prompts can help with portion sizes. Your serving of meat, fish, or chicken ought to be the size of a deck of cards, and a large portion of a cup of crushed potato, rice, or pasta is about the size of a customary light. You can fool your cerebrum into believing it's a more significant portion by serving your meals on little plates or in bowls. If you don't feel fulfilled at the end of a meal, include increasingly verdant greens or adjust the meal with fruit.

Take as much time as necessary. It's imperative to back off and consider food sustenance as opposed to only something to swallow down in the middle of gatherings or while in transit to get the children. It takes a couple of moments for your cerebrum to tell your body that it has had enough food, so eat gradually and quit eating before you feel full.

Eat with others at whatever point conceivable. Eating alone, particularly before the TV or PC, regularly prompts mindless overeating.

Breaking points nibble foods in the home. Be cautious about the foods you keep within reach. It's harder to eat with some restraint if you have unhealthy tidbits and treats right to go. Instead, encircle yourself with healthy choices, and when you're prepared to compensate yourself with a unique treat, go out and get it.

Control enthusiastic eating. We don't always eat just to fulfill hunger. A large number of us additionally go to food to assuage pressure or adapt to upsetting feelings, for example, bitterness, depression, or fatigue. But, by learning healthier ways to oversee stress and feelings, you can regain control over the food you eat and your feelings.

CHAPTER THIRTEEN: MINDFULNESS DIET

Like yoga, healthful eating habits are framed by expectation and practice. Follow this examination sponsored plan to build up your generally adjusted, feasible relationship with food yet.

As an individual who has ever attempted another diet knows, it's anything but difficult to focus on a healthy-eating plan—and significantly simpler to lose steam or self-discipline and discard your purpose following half a month or even days. That is because the greater part of us don't give our new healthy habits the time and consideration they need to get programmed.

A mindful methodology can help you get a charge out of the way toward framing a healthy eating habit, regardless of whether your goal is to pick veggies over refined carbs to get thinner, to back off to appreciate mealtime, or to wipe out meat to coordinate your morals. "Mindfulness helps decline the exertion that people experience in making changes. It appears to help associate us to all the more remarkable ways to change those old neural pathways that are genuinely carved into the mind, and work to discover and make new ones to reinforce."

The accompanying arrangement will assist you with setting genuine desires for the length needed to roll out an enduring improvement, while slowly fusing Mindfulness rehearses, keen food choices, and more delight into every meal.

Focusing on the moment-to-moment experience of eating can help you improve your diet, oversee food longings, and even get in shape. Here's how to begin eating mindfully.

What is mindful eating?

Mindful eating keeps up an in-the-moment familiarity with the food and drink you put into your body, watching as opposed to deciding how the food causes you to feel and the signs your body sends about taste, fulfillment, and totality. Mindful eating expects you just to recognize and acknowledge the feelings, considerations, and substantial sensations you watch— and can reach out to the way toward purchasing, getting ready, and serving your food just as expending it.

For a considerable lot of us, our bustling lives make mealtimes hurried undertakings, or we end up eating in the vehicle driving to work, at the work area before a PC screen, or left on the lounge chair sitting in front of the TV. We eat mindlessly, scooping food down whether or not we're as yet eager or not. We regularly eat for reasons other than hunger—to fulfill enthusiastic needs, to assuage pressure, or adapt to undesirable feelings, for example, pity, tension, depression, or weariness. Mindful eating is something contrary to this sort of unhealthy "mindless" eating.

Mindful eating isn't tied in with being great, always eating the right things, or never permitting yourself to eat in a hurry again. Furthermore, it's not tied in with setting up strict principles for what number of calories you can eat or which foods you need to include or maintain a strategic distance from in your diet. Or maybe it's tied in with centering every one of your faculties and being available as you shop, cook, serve, and eat your food. While mindfulness isn't for everybody, numerous people find that by eating along these lines, in any event, for only a couple of meals seven days, you can turn out to be more receptive to your body. This can help you abstain from overeating and make it simpler to change your dietary habits to improve things and appreciate the improved mental and physical prosperity that accompanies a healthier diet.

Advantages of mindful eating

By giving close consideration to how you feel as you eat—the surface and tastes of every significant piece, your body's yearning, and totality signals, how different foods influence your energy and state of mind—you can figure out how to appreciate both your food and the experience of eating. Being mindful of the food you eat can advance better processing, keep you full with less food, and impact more intelligent choices about what you eat later on. It can likewise assist you with freeing yourself from unhealthy habits around food and eating.

Eating mindfully can push you to:

- Slow down and enjoy a reprieve from the hurrying around of your day, facilitating pressure and nervousness.
- Look at and change your relationship with food—helping you, for instance, to notice when you go to food for reasons other than hunger.
- Get more noteworthy delight from the food you eat, as you figure out how to back off and all the more completely value your meals and tidbits.
- Settle on healthier choices about what you eat by concentrating on how each kind of food causes you to feel in the wake of eating it.
- Improve your processing by eating more slowly.
- Feel fuller sooner and by eating less food.
- Make a more prominent association with where your food originates from, how it's delivered, and the journey it's taken to your plate.
- Eat in a healthier, progressively adjusted way.

The most effective method to rehearse mindful eating

To rehearse mindfulness, you need to take an interest in an activity with all-out mindfulness. On account of mindful eating, it's essential to eat with all your consideration as opposed to on "programmed pilot" or while you're perusing, taking a gander at your telephone, sitting in front of the TV, daydreaming, or arranging what you're doing later. At the point when your consideration strays, tenderly take it back to your food and the experience of cooking, serving, and eating.

Have a go at rehearsing mindful eating for short, five-minute spans from the start and steadily developing from that point. Furthermore, recollect: you can start mindful eating when you're making your shopping rundown or perusing the menu at an eatery. Cautiously evaluate everything you add to your rundown or browse the list.

Start by taking a couple of full breaths and considering the health estimation of each different bit of food. While nourishment specialists ceaselessly banter precisely which foods are "healthy" and which are not, the best dependable guideline is to eat food that is as close as conceivable to the way nature made it.

Utilize every one of your faculties while you're shopping, cooking, serving, and eating your food. How do different foods look, smell, and feel as you hack? How would they sound as they're being cooked? How would they taste as you eat?

Be interested and mention objective facts about yourself, just as the food you're going to eat. Notice how you're sitting; sit with a high stance; however, stay relaxed. Recognize your environmental factors yet figure out how to block them out. Concentrating on what's happening around, you may divert from your procedure of eating and detract from the experience.

Tune into your yearning: How hungry, right? You need to get together when you're eager but not greedy in the wake of skipping meals. Realize what your expectations are in eating this specific meal. Is it true that you are eating because you're really hungry, or is it that you're exhausted, need an interruption, or believe it's what you ought to do?

With the food before you, pause for a minute to welcome it—and any people you're imparting the meal too—before eating. Focus on the surfaces, shapes, hues, and scents of the food. What responses do you have to the food, and how do the scents cause you to feel?

Take a nibble, and notice how it feels in your mouth. How might you portray the surface at this point? Attempt to identify all the fixings, all the different flavors. Bite completely and notice how you bite and what that feels like.

Concentrate on how your experience shifts from moment to moment. Do you feel yourself getting full? Is it accurate to say that you are fulfilled? Take as much time as is needed, remain present, and don't surge the experience.

Put your utensils down between chomps. Set aside some effort to consider how you feel—eager, satisfied—before getting your utensils again. Tune in to your stomach, not your plate. Realize when you're full and quit eating.

Give appreciation and think about where this food originated from, the plants or creatures included, and all the people it took to ship the food and bring it onto your plate. Being progressively mindful about the starting points of our food can help all of us make smarter and increasingly manageable choices.

Keep on eating gradually as you talk with your eating colleagues, paying close attention to your body's signals of fullness. If eating alone, attempt to stay present to the experience of devouring the meal.

Fitting mindful eating into your life

For the vast majority of us, it's ridiculous to figure we can be mindful of each nibble or even for each meal we eat. The weights of work and family sometimes mean you're compelled to eat in a hurry or have just a constrained window to eat something or hazard going hungry for the remainder of the day. Be that as it may, even when you can't cling to a cruel mindful eating practice, you can, in any case, abstain from eating mindlessly and disregarding your body's signals.

Maybe you can take a couple of full breaths before eating a meal or tidbit to unobtrusively consider what you're going to place into your body. Is it accurate to say that you are eating in the light of craving signals, or would you say you are eating because of an emotional sign? Perhaps you're exhausted or on edge or desolate? Also, would you say you are eating food that is healthfully sound, or would you say you are eating emotionally soothing food? Even if you need to eat at your work area, for instance, would you be able to take a couple of seconds to focus all your attention on your food instead of performing various tasks or being diverted by your PC or telephone?

Consider mindful eating like exercise: every piece tallies. The more you can never really down, focus exclusively on the way toward eating, and tune in to your body, the more prominent satisfaction you'll encounter from your food and the more prominent control you'll have over your eating regimen and nourishment habits.

Changing from mindless to mindful eating

Eating on autopilot or while performing multiple tasks (driving, working, perusing, staring at the TV, etc.)	Focusing all your attention on your food and the experience of eating.
Eating until all the food has gone; disregarding your body's signals of fullness.	Listening to your body's signals and eating just until you're full.

Eating to fill an emotional void (because you're stressed, desolate, miserable, or exhausted, for example)	Eating just to fulfill the physical appetite.
Eating garbage or solace food.	Eating healthfully solid meals and bites.
Eating food as fast as possible.	Eating gradually, relishing each chomp.

Utilizing mindfulness to investigate your relationship with food

Regardless of whether you're mindful of it or not, food significantly affects your prosperity. It can affect how you feel genuinely, how you react emotionally, and how you oversee intellectually. It can help your energy and viewpoint, or it can deplete your assets and make you feel weary, ill-humored, and discouraged.

We, as a whole, realize that we should eat less sugar and prepare foods and more soil products. Be that as it may, if basically knowing the "rules" of proper dieting was sufficient, none of us would be overweight or snared on low-quality nourishment. At the point when you eat mindfully and turn out to be more sensitive to your body, in any case, you can begin to feel how different foods affect you genuinely, intellectually, and emotionally. What's more, that can make it a lot simpler to make the change to more beneficial food choices. For instance, when you understand that the sugary nibble you need when you're worn out or discouraged really leaves you feeling even more regrettable, it's simpler to deal with those desires and decide on a more advantageous bite that helps your energy and state of mind.

A considerable lot of us just indeed pay attention to how food affects us when it makes us truly sick. The inquiry we ought to present isn't, "Does my food make me wiped out?" but instead, "How well does it make me feel?" at the end of the day, how much better do you feel in the wake of eating? What amount more energy and excitement do you have after a meal or tidbit?

How does your food make you feel?

To thoroughly investigate your relationship with food, it's essential to get mindful of how different foods make you feel. How would you feel after you swallow the food? How would you feel quickly, in 60 minutes, or a few hours after eating? How would you think by and large for the day?

To begin following the connection between what you eat and how it affects you, attempt the accompanying exercise:

Following the connection between food and feeling

Eat in your standard way. Select the foods, sums, and the times for eating that you ordinarily do, just currently add mindfulness to what you are doing.

Track all that you eat, including snacks and snacks between meals. Try not to mess with yourself—you won't recollect everything unless you record everything or track it in an application!

Pay attention to your feelings—physical and emotional—five minutes after you have eaten; one hour after you have eaten; a few hours after you have eaten.

Notice if there has been a shift or change as the consequence of eating. Improve or more regrettable than before you ate? Do you feel invigorated or tired? Alert or lazy?

Keeping a record on your telephone or in a note pad can elevate your attention to how the meals and snacks you eat affect your state of mind and prosperity.

Exploring different avenues regarding different food combinations

When you're ready to associate your food choices to your physical and mental prosperity, the procedure of food determination turns into a matter of carefully tuning in to your own body. For instance, you may find that when you eat starches, you feel heavy and torpid for a considerable length of time. In this manner, carb-heavy meals become something you attempt to dodge.

Different foods affect every one of us differently, as indicated by elements such as hereditary qualities and lifestyle. The best way to honestly know how different foods and combinations of food will affect you is through experimentation. Consider it like choosing whether or not to take a specific nutrient or supplement. The way you feel when you take the nutrient or supplement will frequently reveal to you whether your body needs it.

The accompanying exercise can assist you in finding how different food combinations and amounts affect your prosperity:

Blending and coordinating different foods

Start to explore different avenues regarding your food:

- Have a go at eating less food more regularly, or less food, period.
- If you're a meat-eater, go through a few days barring meat from your eating routine.
- Or, on the other hand, maybe prohibit red meat, but incorporate chicken and fish.

- Expel certain foods from your eating routine: salt, sugar, espresso, or bread, for instance, and perceive how this affects how you feel.
- Play with food combinations. Take a stab at eating exclusively starch meals, protein meals, natural product meals, or vegetable meals.
- Track everything you see in yourself as you explore different avenues regarding your eating habits. The inquiry you're attempting to answer is: "Which eating designs add to the nature of my life, and which degrade?"
- Keep exploring different avenues regarding different sorts, combinations, and measures of food for half a month, following how you feel intellectually, genuinely, and emotionally.

Eating to fill a void versus eating to improve prosperity

While eating without a doubt affects how you feel, it's also self-evident how you think affects what, when, and the amount you eat. A significant number of us now and again botch feelings of nervousness, stress, depression, or weariness for cravings for food and use food trying to adapt to these feelings. The distress you feel reminds you that you need something and fill a void in your life. That void could be a superior relationship, an even more satisfying activity, or a profound need. At the point when you consistently attempt to fill that void with food, though, you definitely neglect your genuine appetites.

As you practice mindful eating and your mindfulness develops, you'll become mindful of how regularly your food utilization has nothing to do with physical craving. Everything to do with filling an emotional need. As you plunk down to eat, ask yourself, "What am I hungry for?" Do you need that "small something to snack on" because you're genuinely eager or for another explanation? Filling and soaking yourself with food can help cover what you're incredibly hungry for, however, just for a brief timeframe. And afterward, the genuine appetite or need will return.

Pick your mindful eating homework.

1. Try taking the initial four tastes of some hot tea or espresso with full attention?

2. If you are perusing and eating, take a stab at exchanging these exercises, not doing both on the double? Peruse a page; at that point, put the book down, eat a couple of nibbles, and relish the preferences, at that point, read another page.

3. At family meals, you may approach everybody to eat peacefully for the initial five minutes, contemplating the numerous people who carried the food to your plates.

4. Try eating one meal seven days mindfully, alone and peacefully. Be inventive. For instance, would you be able to have lunch behind a shut office entryway, or even alone in our vehicle?

CHAPTER FOURTEEN: GOAL SETTING AFFIRMATIONS

HOW AFFIRMATIONS CAN BE EMPLOYED IN DAILY LIFE

Affirmations can fill in as a significant instrument for staying on target and fighting off feelings of demoralization. To utilize the past model, an affirmation to address tension or cynicism around weight concerns could be, "Every day, I am one bit nearer to achieving my most advantageous weight." If the negative self-talk is progressively summed up or self-basic, one may make an affirmation, for example, "I band together with my body in keeping myself well." An affirmation that is counter to negative feelings or convictions identified with exercise is, "It feels great to eat well and move my body."

Once more, a gainful affirmation is correctly identified with a positive goal, something contrary to what the negative self-talk says, and causes one to envision a successful result.

AFFIRMATIONS PRESENT AND FUTURE

Although affirmations are usually expressed in the current state (to encourage a feeling of these announcements previously being valid), asserting proclamations can likewise be joined with guided or self-guided symbolism to focus on future success. This method is really utilized in trance and self-trance and is referred to as "future movement." Future movement symbolism includes creating the multisensory experience of being at that time when one has achieved a future goal, even though the real symbolism is occurring within oneself, right now.

HOW AFFIRMATIONS WORK

Although creating affirmations can be clear, ongoing exploration has discovered affirmations adequately increment feelings of prosperity and improve the probability of using sound judgment. As you've presumably seen, when under stress, many people are increasingly helpless against self-uncertainty or feeling overwhelmed all in all. Affirmations seem to work by reminding us of individual assets past what we notice when we are debilitated. Relatedly, affirmations appear to assist us with reflecting on our guiding principle and draw upon the positive individual encounters we've had.

AFFIRMATIONS AND THE BRAIN

A few different cerebrum locales are thought to be associated with the advantages seen identified by taking part in affirmations. For instance, in past examinations, the ventral striatum and the ventral average prefrontal cortex have been connected to allocating a positive incentive to something (for example, achieving a goal) and survey it as a prize. Expanded movement in the average prefrontal cortex and back cingulate cortex have been connected to focusing on one's very own qualities. Also, self-affirmations may work to a limited extent by connecting with the front cingulate cortex and the ventrolateral prefrontal cortex to manage emotions (fighting off negative emotions, or staying progressively objective) when confronted with difficult situations.

We, as a whole, have our stages when negative and harmful feelings inundate us. We feel every one of our endeavors is squandered.

This transpired some time back, I was feeling overwhelmed, stressed, and simply miserable.

I had zero motivation to work for quite a long time together.

There were things which didn't go as arranged, leaving me sad.

Thankfully, I understood something needed to change. I needed to change. My satisfaction is most extremely critical to me, and I can never settle on this.

There was no chance I would let pessimism overwhelm me.

I had an ambiguous thought regarding self-affirmations; however, I indeed took rehearsing it during that difficult time.

These are some positive affirmations that helped me to skip back.

What are self-affirmations?

Self-Affirmations are your catchphrases or articulations that you express for motivation, certainty, and motivation.

Studies have indicated that self-affirmations help you to focus and focus better on your goals.

How to rehearse it?

There are no firm guidelines. You can express these announcements at whatever point you feel low.

You can rehash these announcements consistently, any day at a specific time, or at whatever point you wish.

Yet, if you ask me, I will desire to first to have faith in these affirmations before repeating.

If you don't have confidence in affirmations, these will

be simply words or some jibber-jabber that you rehashed.

Have confidence in what you are stating and simply observe the difference.

With respect to rehearsing, it might appear to be odd from the outset to say for all to hear; however, it helps if your ear can hear you talk these sentences.

So you don't generally need to yell yet state it noisy enough for you to hear it.

Self-affirmations for motivation and goal-setting

I grasp myself fully and completely.

This is my standard number one in life. I am finished with what others consider me.

Some time ago, I was easily affected by everyone's opinion of me.

It made a difference to me an extraordinary arrangement so much that it affected my psychological harmony. I was furious and bothered quite often.

There was an excessive number of people in my life, and genuinely it felt somewhat swarmed.

So when I chose to remove all negative and poisonous people, my life improved like enchantment.

Today I have fewer people, yet they are astonishing and my most grounded mainstays of help.

If you identify with this, let me disclose to you I hear you, I get you, and this is the explanation in all seriousness needn't bother with approval from anybody.

Above all, for what reason do you need approval from anybody? Grasp yourself as well as other people will tail you.

How often you were dismal because your Instagram likes were not many or when somebody didn't commend you enough or the times you adjusted yourself to fit into a specific group?

Consider it!

If you feel demotivated by what others state, perhaps it's time to move away from such people.

Affirmations for Motivation

I am propelled and roused.

At the point when you are demotivated, recollect it's only a stage, a testing time.

However, time changes, and it possibly shows signs of improvement when you have seen you are more awful.

So better days are indeed ahead; you simply need to trust in yourself and move to continue onward.

It is appropriately said life is an exciting ride, so there are good days and bad days.

It is said bad days are essential to acknowledge good times.

I am benefiting as much as possible from this beautiful day.

This basic expression is so ground-breaking when you understand its profundity.

Each day brings some new chance. It allows you to change yourself.

It allows you to make something new.

At the point when you are hindered, and you find positively no motivation to work, rehash this line.

Consider how best you can live this day. What can you do another way today?

You can make every single day the greatest day of your life.

Value every day, and be appreciative you are living.

I am pleased with myself.

Is it true that you are pleased with yourself?

Is it true that you are pleased with how far you have come and the amount you have achieved? No?

You ought to reflect where you began and where you stand now.

Consider each achievement you have achieved, how you took care of each issue.

Comprehend your self-esteem and offer credit to yourself where it's expected.

You endure, and that one straightforward reality is so persuasive.

My life is getting down to business beautifully.

What's more, trust me, everything eventually takes care of business.

My mix-ups just make me better.

Everybody makes botches, and that is alright. Accept each mix-up as an expectation to absorb information.

Your mix-ups will make just you better and increasingly experienced.

Rather than agonizing over slip-ups, acknowledge it and proceed onward.

I am special.

The current total populace is more than 7 billion, and every person in this world is brought into the world with an interesting personality.

Isn't it an explanation enough to celebrate?

There is, after all, nobody very like you in this whole world. Consider that phenomenal thought.

I am giving my best at each second.

This self-affirmation is for those minutes when you feel overwhelmed by stuff.

Life can be difficult even on ordinary days. Simply make sure to continue breathing.

At the point when I feel overwhelmed, there is only one thing I do – rest.

I simply take a good long rest, and when I wake up, I feel much improved.

I am gaining inconceivable ground everyday.

Difficulties are frustrating; however, when you quit something because of not many misfortunes, that is even more harming.

Rather than feeling demotivated, work more earnestly.

At the point when you continue advancing despite difficulties, it implies you are destined for success and genuinely inspired to achieve your goals.

I am full of positive energy.

Do you get the feeling that a few spots are flawless to

such an extent that you never need to leave?

Your life is much the same as that. We all pull in positive and negative energies.

There are a few people you feel so good around them, while there are some who radiate a negative vibe.

The sort of energies you pull in will make you the kind of individual you need to be.

I am higher than my feelings of trepidation.

This affirmation will give you the boldness to push ahead and face difficulties head-on.

It will assist you with getting out of your customary range of familiarity, which you thoroughly should.

I am creating an astonishing life for myself.

You have the ability to make an extraordinarily beautiful life for yourself.

A life you totally merit. In particular, you can do it; you just need to accept it.

Half of your work is done if you just have faith in yourself.

I am my biggest cheerleader.

Indeed sweetheart! You do your thing.

Be your biggest cheerleader, and change that tide.

Even when others don't pull for you, you need to be your most grounded help.

I make choices rapidly.

There will be occasions when others may question your choices; however, if you feel it in your gut that it's the correct choice, you should take it.

Likewise, it may be the case that not every one of your choices may bear similar outcomes, and it is totally alright.

So don't lament any choice you make, instead consider it a venturing stone to success.

My dangers pay off and advance my business

This is significant if you have your own endeavor.

You should be happy to face challenges.

Try not to be apprehensive when you need to take a less secure way.

If you heed your gut feelings, you will not fizzle.

I am sure.

Be positive about your skin; there is nothing more beautiful than a sure individual, not over-keen, not presumption, but rather a calm certainty radiating from your emanation.

I will give my 100% and then some.

Success requests difficult work. So give your 100% and more if you need to be successful.

There are times you will feel like quitting any pretense of bailing.

Yet, trust in yourself during those times, hold that jaw up and push forward.

I set out to be different.

Relatively few people can set out to be different, be that individual who dares, makes a personality, and stands separated from the group.

I am beautiful.

There are such huge numbers of us who are perpetually discontent with the way we look.

We want to be better, higher. Yet, flawlessness is a figment.

So express this to yourself each day until you trust it.

I am loaded up with wealth.

There is a familiar axiom, "grumble less, and you will pick up."

Henceforth focus on the good things in your life. Think about how satisfying your life is.

I am encircled by affection, chuckling, and inspiration.

Ponder each one of those people who have had a positive effect on your life.

Is it accurate to say that you are unsettled to have them?

At the point when you feel demotivated, recollect those people who made you chuckle, who love you.

AFFIRMATIONS TO ACHIEVE YOUR GOALS

I will achieve more goals quickly.

Consistently I make a move to achieve my goals.

My mind is focused on completing things.

It is simple for me to achieve my goals.

I am resolved to achieve my goals.

Nothing will prevent me from achieving my goals.

I have confidence in myself and my goals

I am figuring out how to confide in myself to achieve my goals.

I am 100% dedicated to making my goals a reality.

I have the force and capacity to achieve my goals.

I make a move towards my goals consistently.

I realize that anything is conceivable when I make a move.

I realize that I can achieve anything I set out to do

I see steady outcomes of my actions.

I am propelled and invigorated to achieve my goals.

Consistently, I am ever nearer to achieving my goals.

I am easily ready to discover any assets I require to achieve my goals.

I appreciate making a move to make my goal a reality.

I am ready to achieve anything I set my focus on

I realize that I will achieve my goal.

I can do this, and I will!

AFFIRMATIONS TO ACHIEVE SUCCESS

I can achieve anything I set my focus on.

Achieving success comes easily and naturally to me.

Being successful feels good, and I am glad for my

success.

There is nothing that can prevent me from achieving success.

I have confidence in my capacities to achieve success and riches.

Success is my claim.

AFFIRMATIONS TO GET MORE DONE

I appreciate being profitable.

I am profitable in all regions.

Consistently I am completing things ease.

I love completing my assignments on time.

I am turning out to be increasingly beneficial every day.

People consider me to be an exceptionally beneficial individual.

Nothing can prevent me from completing things.

AFFIRMATIONS TO STAY FOCUSED

I think that it's simple to stay focused on my undertakings.

Nothing can occupy me from completing my activity.

Being focused and inspired comes easily to me.

I appreciate being focused on my activity.

I am completely calm, focused, and persuaded to would anything I like to.

I am laser-focused to complete more.

AFFIRMATIONS TO DEVELOP GOOD HABITS

Every day I am working on developing better habits.

Good habits make my life simpler.

Having good and reliable habits is valuable to me.

I think that it's simple to develop good habits.

I love staying focused on my good habits.

Good habits keep me focused on achieving my goals.

AFFIRMATIONS TO STOP PROCRASTINATING

I appreciate being proactive and profitable.

I love getting an encouraging start and completing

things on time.

Completing things has become my preferred thing.

Being a practitioner falls into place without any issues for me.

I can easily assume responsibility and change something I don't care for.

Nothing will hinder me from making a move today.

CHAPTER FIFTEEN: SELF-CONTROL AFFIRMATIONS

Do you realize how there's each one of those platitudes about taking care of your mind and your thoughts molding your life and all that yadda? I've thought that its everything to be exceptionally evident recently as much as I flinch at the triteness of certain statements out there. Sometimes those silly ones are simply so darn precise.

Yet, I'm attempting to move beyond the cliché perspective and understand that the entirety of our thoughts truly has such a great amount of impact on our lives. It resembles when you're feeling good, you emanate so much energy, and you feel like nothing can hinder that. Your positive thoughts pull in even increasingly positive thoughts, and progressively positive things continue transpiring.

Something very similar applies when you're feeling bad. Your mind tops off with cynicism. It turns out to be almost difficult to see the good in anything, and you drag every other person down with you. Those negative thoughts make even greater pessimism around you to where it feels like everything is turning out badly, and nothing is in your control.

So I understand that it's so imperative to break that cycle before it gets that far. It additionally assists in preventing those feelings inside and out.

One compelling way to do that is through positive affirmations. I always hear that it's more impressive to state them for all to hear, however even reminding yourself in your own head is useful. This rundown of affirmations is extremely incredible for getting yourself through difficult times.

For the greatest outcomes, you should work on utilizing affirmations in any event twice every day. For this situation, we likewise exhort that you retain a couple of you can approach in difficult situations when you feel yourself losing emotional control. Focus on your breathing, rehash your picked affirmations, discharge any pressure in your body, and you WILL recover control over yourself.

In time these positive affirmations will assist you with taking a few to get back some composure on your emotions, and you will think that it's simpler and simpler to calm yourself down and locate your middle. Eventually, you will turn out to be more naturally calm in stressful situations, more in control of outrage and stress, and just by and large more in control of yourself and your emotions in all situations.

Here they are, pick a not many that truly address you

and make them your own. With devotion and everyday practice, you will figure out how to control your emotions for the last time!

Whatever didn't complete yesterday or needs to complete today can hang tight until further notice.

I am focused on watching out for my needs, intellectually, profoundly, and emotionally.

It's alright for me to take the time that is important to work on me.

I will travel during this time with a feeling of appreciation.

I am appreciative for another chance to be my best self.

I am mindful and on top of my qualities and shortcomings.

Today I will be purposeful about setting up limits and constraining distractions so I can achieve today's goals.

I am in control of how I utilize my time. Today I will get out from under bad habits.

I have the willpower to focus on coordinating my conduct with my wants for life I need to assemble.

I do what I state I will do. At the point when I declare, I will do it.

I achieve my undertakings and always finish.

I always give my best at whatever I do.

I work on a feeling of greatness.

I am efficient in each aspect of my life.

I have the willpower to work through as well as around any difficulties the day may bring.

I can depend on myself to do what I need to do and hit my objectives.

I will trust in the Lord to reinforce me in any region that I may miss the mark.

I am focused on the reason God is calling me to and to satisfying the fate He has for me.

I have the order to go to Him first in the petition, so I am adjusting my goals to His guarantees for my life.

Every one of my choices is in concurrence with my wants.

Every one of my habits is under my complete control.

Consistently I improve my willpower through steady practice.

Consistently my willpower gets more grounded.

Each snapshot of consistently, I am turning out to be increasingly trained.

Practicing discretion gives me a tremendous feeling of achievement.

I recognize my resistance and push ahead anyway.

I always do what I state I will do. My statement is the law.

I always finish.

I always set forth my earnest attempts into everything I do.

I am over all allurements.

I am fully in control of all that I do.

I am accountable for my practices and actions.

I am accountable for my life.

I am in complete control of my thoughts, my actions, and my life.

I am in complete control of what I do in my life.

I am in complete control over my past impairing habits.

I am currently in control of everything I state and do.

I am the chief of my life.

I am the ace of my life.

I am efficient in each aspect of my life.

I will take the necessary steps.

I apply my willpower to improving my character and capacities.

I make significant decisions in my life.

I can rely on myself to do what I need to do.

I ultimately control the words and habits in my life.

I control all motivations in my life.

I control the heading of my thoughts.

I hunger for just that which I have made my goal.

I direct my self-discipline to focus on the vision of what I need with the confidence that it is as of now mine.

I easily resist all urges that endanger my goals.

I easily resist anything that endeavors to divert me from my way.

I exercise poise in all that I do.

I face all difficulties with sharp resolve.

AFFIRMATIONS FOR DISCIPLINE

I make good choices.

I finish my duties.

I offer 100% to everything I do.

I am the Master of my fate.

I never get diverted.

I utilize my time astutely.

I have an abundance of energy.

I make results.

I am profoundly sorted out and taught.

I am in control of my thoughts, choices, and actions.

I set and achieve goals efficiently.

I complete a great deal.

I have a dependable and trained mind.

I carry on with my life with laser focus.

Consistently my willpower gets more grounded through my habits.

I make choices that assist me in achieving my goals.

I never surrender.

I appreciate difficult work and misfortune.

I have the self-control of a zen ace.

I finish all undertakings that I start.

I focus all my energy and will on what I realize must be finished.

I focus my thoughts and actions just on achieving my goals.

I have bottomless oomph and staying power.

I have all the resolve I need to.

I have all the resolve I need to understand my goals.

I have all the resolve I need to succeed.

I have an iron will with regards to working on my goals.

I have complete control over my actions.

I have complete control over my habits.

I have fantastic restraint.

I have the order essential to defeat any test.

I have the ability to pick my thoughts and actions.

I have the ability to keep on target.

I have the self-control required to be a victor.

I have the quality of mind to control my actions.

I have the quality of will to stay on the way I have

picked.

I have the willpower and determination to defeat all impediments.

I have complete control over my actions and practices.

I have enduring assurance and willpower.

I have unwavering resolve and constancy.

I respect all choices in my life with ardent resolve.

I keep my eyes on what I need, and this engages my will.

I realize that difficulties will pass and that I will be triumphant.

I realize that it is always too early to stop.

I realize that willpower improves with exercise.

I never debilitate my will by surrendering or surrendering.

I just acknowledge those urges that help my wants.

I drive forward with hopefulness and excitement.

I endure and continue – regardless.

I have incredible inward quality and guts.

I proceed towards my goals, regardless.

I will not permit any thoughts or actions to subvert my motivation.

I resist all enticements as they emerge.

I resolve all issues in my life with resolute resolve.

I assume absolute liability for every one of my choices and actions.

I utilize my unwavering resolve to keep myself on target.

I utilize my willpower to focus my thoughts on my motivation and my goals.

My astounding discretion keeps me on target with my goals.

My longing to succeed is back by a will of iron.

My massive poise lifts my certainty and confidence.

My staggering poise guarantees that I always stay on target.

My thoughts and actions are entirely heavily influenced by me.

My unwavering resolve bolsters all that I do.

My will is almighty.

My will is incredible.

My will is reliable and incredible.

My willpower is always more grounded than any allurement I experience.

My willpower is persistent.

My willpower is solid because I realize what I need and prop up until I succeed.

My willpower is unfaltering.

My assertion is the law.

Nothing can prevent me from achieving.

Nothing can prevent me from achieving my goals.

Nothing can prevent me from arriving at my goals.

Having incredible willpower is one of the top needs in my life, and I practice this feeling each day.

Poise incredibly raises my feeling of certainty and confidence.

The more I exercise my willpower, the more grounded it becomes.

Today I favor my being with endless willpower.

Today I favor my being with boundless resolve.

Today I decide to assume complete responsibility for my

life.

Whatever I choose to do becomes unquestionable law in my life.

When hard times arise, I get moving.

Willpower is a habit that I support each day.

With each breath I take, I am bringing increasingly more control into my life.

Current state Affirmations

I am in control of my emotions.

I am always focused and calm.

I always keep control of myself consistently.

My mind is focused, clear, and sensible.

I stay calm in stressful situations.

I am trustworthy and in control.

I am ready to manage stressful situations in a controlled way.

I feel emotions without losing control.

I manage an abundance of emotions in a positive way.

My emotions are leveled out consistently.

Future Tense Affirmations

I will resist the urge to panic.

I will control my emotions.

I am changing into somebody who is naturally calm and gathered.

Others are starting to see how in control of myself I am

I feel that it's simpler to calm myself down

I am overseeing my emotions as time passes.

Controlling my emotions is getting simpler and simpler.

I am starting to think consistently, even in stressful situations.

Stressful situations are getting simpler to manage.

I will manage my emotions in a positive style.

Normal Affirmations

Controlling my emotions is simple for me.

Feeling calm is typical for me.

I can easily deal with my emotions.

I can think plainly, even in difficult and tense situations.

My mind is always calm, explicit, and legitimate

Directing my emotions is something I simply do naturally.

I can feel emotions without turning wild.

Controlling my emotions will improve my life.

Others will look to me as somebody who tries to avoid panicking in stressful situations.

I have the ability to control my emotions completely

CHAPTER SIXTEEN: EXERCISE MOTIVATION

Are there days when you experience difficulty getting propelled to exercise even though you know it's keen for your heart? You're not the only one. Particularly during the initial three or four months of another exercise program, it very well may be intellectually difficult to continue moving.

Calorie counters who kept a food journal lost twice as much weight as the individuals who kept no records. In any case, while keeping a diary considers you progressively responsible for how you treat your body, adhering to a fitness routine is different from adhering to proper dieting daily schedule.

If it were anything but difficult to stay roused to work out, at that point, we'd all have rock-hard abs. Oh, the drive to get up for an early morning sweat meeting is tricky, aside from those irresistibly positive and enthusiastic fitness coaches and teachers—or so you thought. Even they need some consolation sometimes.

It's simple (and even significant, as a major aspect of a goal-setting procedure) to make intends to exercise. It's the finish that sometimes gets people made up for a lost time. That is the place motivation comes in. It provides reason and guidance to your conduct, giving the inside push you need to conquer pardons and begin. Sadly, sometimes it abandons you right when you need it most.

The Source of Motivation

For competitors, motivation to exercise may originate from the craving to contend and win. For different exercises, it might originate from a desire to be solid or live longer for their children. For some, getting more fit is the goal.

A significant number of us accept motivation will come to us if we stand by sufficiently long: Someday, we'll wake up lastly need to exercise. Motivation is something we can and need to make for ourselves.

Utilize the accompanying components to make your own motivation, and you'll see it simpler to stay with your workouts. At that point, you'll begin seeing the aftereffects of your endeavors, which may help fuel your will to continue onward.

Take another class

Your preferred educators are extraordinary instructors; however, they're still understudies, as well.

Group fitness is something other than a workout; however, a chance to perceive what different teachers are doing and get new thoughts. "We're still buyers of group fitness."

Treat yourself consistently

To stay on target with a solid, adjusted eating routine. "If I permit myself a treat, I'm way more reluctant to enjoy or gorge. One glass of wine is great, however, an entire container? Wrecking."

This savvy eating methodology is the explanation numerous specialists state stylish or prohibitive eating regimens just don't work. You wind up longing for oneself prohibited food even progressively, expanding your chances of gorging or tumbling off the cart completely.

Siphon up the jams

Music can be an inconceivably amazing disposition supporter. Research has demonstrated that tuning in to glad or tragic music can very modify the way you see the world—ground-breaking stuff!

"Regardless of what the situation is—an early reminder, runs on the treadmill, or simply having a life second, music takes me back to me."

Give yourself a motivational speech

Regardless of whether it's a relative's uplifting statements that have stayed with you or verses from a natural tune, keeping a mantra, catchphrase, or maxim helpful when you need an increase in certainty or assurance can work ponders.

It's just "We should go! I have this." "If I'm going into a gathering, or absolutely biting the dust during a workout meeting, I'll state it [to myself]."

Plan a post-workout meal

Having a portion of food in mind for your post-workout grub will propel you to smash your perspiration meeting. "It's something I get amped up for." That stated, don't try too hard—recall these tips for maintaining a strategic distance from a post-workout gorge.

Associate with companions

A workout mate considers you responsible for the time and exertion you put into your workouts—research demonstrates it. Also, associating as you sweat can make exercise progressively fun.

"I love welcoming my companions to go along with me in class, as well. The more people I need to anticipate, the more I feel spurred to be at the highest point of my game."

Work on being mindful

The craft of being at the time, shutting out all the outside day-to-day stressors that can disrupt the general

flow is sometimes more difficult than one might expect,
Where your mind goes, your energy goes with it."

Encircle yourself with positive people

It's ideal for encircling yourself with companions who have comparative interests; it's similarly as essential to be with people who are doing things you need to do. If you see others living healthfully, those actions could become habits for you, as well.

"If you have somebody helping you to stay predictable, it's a distinct advantage."

Tune in to your body

Your body could be disclosed to you things you might not have any desire to hear. "So I glance around at others at the exercise center or in class and let myself know if they can do it, so can I."

Different times though, your body may be cautioning you to stop. "There's nothing amiss with taking a break, and there's nothing less persuading than a physical issue. If my body feels excessively exhausted, or I feel uneasiness in my muscles or joints, I ease off. Staying protected and sound takes into consideration life span, and that is truly what it's everything about."

Get in those means for the afternoon

You pursued turn class just to acknowledge it was in the

area across town. Rather than fearing the drive, make good utilization of that time! "Sometimes, to get roused for class, I constrain myself to run, walk, or bicycle there as opposed to accepting the subway as a way to get my blood streaming and endorphins up."

Studies have indicated that practicing outside (or for this situation, taking the panoramic detour to class) offers extra advantages like improved disposition and, assuming the rainclouds hold back, an additional portion of vitamin D.

Consider what you can achieve at this moment

You may have a bigger goal in mind—dropping pounds, preparing for a long-distance race—however, it's critical to recall all the infant steps it takes to arrive.

Heads up

The floor-to-roof mirrors encompassing most studios are not there to torment you. Without a doubt, you may feel somewhat ungainly while you're getting the hang of an especially testing move, yet glancing in the mirror can help idealize your structure after some time.

The mirror helps show you exactly how hard you are working. "Seeing my muscles work is an enormous inspiration. The better time and fitted I can get my workout garments, the more I can unmistakably observe the goals I'm attempting to achieve—and look good [while] doing it!"

Drink more matcha

If you're not a very remarkable espresso consumer but instead still need a speedy caffeine fix, attempt matcha, a powdered type of green tea. "A matcha green tea latte with almond milk is my go-to. It's my solitary caffeine admission, so I get a flood of energy!"

The focus on matcha has become more brilliant as of late, and for good explanation. Because you are drinking the entire tea leaves (rather than just soaking them), matcha drinks are a more intense wellspring of supplements than conventional teas. Matcha is wealthy in cell reinforcements that may secure against coronary illness and malignant growth, just as help manage glucose and pulse.

"Sometimes, I monitor fitness hashtags on Instagram to perceive what others are doing. Seeing bodies moving and pictures of solidarity spurs me."

Recollect the fact of the matter isn't to contrast yourself with others (everybody's wellbeing excursion and physical make-up is different). Instead, consider what or who moves you to get going and have confidence in yourself and afterward follow educators, mentors, or studios via web-based networking media for some fitspiration. It is anything but an evil plan to follow your preferred magazines.

Consider how you'll feel after

"I work out for my rational soundness, not vanity. Workouts are my treatment. I know if I don't get the chance to discharge those endorphins, I'm not as joyful."

Exercise has for quite some time been appeared to have enduring emotional wellness benefits well after you complete a workout. Action (even only a stroll around the square) is said to reduce stress, help your temperament, and develop confidence. Those great mental impacts ought to be motivation enough to get you up and out.

Be appreciative

It's very simple to become involved with your own issues, dissatisfactions, or ceaseless plan for the day. Yet, you think that it's accommodating to move in the opposite direction from grumblings and consider what she must be grateful for. Remind yourself that you have the essential capacity to move. "Be appreciative that you have two legs that work. Try not to underestimate that."

It's this appreciation that keeps you pushing ahead every day. "I consider people who can't move, and it places everything in context for me."

Go out to shop

They state when you look good, you feel good. Sounds like a reason to go out to shop! What's more, Swan is certainly ready, "I'm not going to mislead anybody, another exercise center outfit gives me motivation. Fresh out of the box new spandex or a stellar games bra is much the same as purchasing the ideal minimal dark dress."

Something other than retail treatment, venturing into fun new workout wear could be only the increase in self-esteem you need to adhere to a weight reduction goal or thorough preparing plan. What's more, further exploration proposes that dressing for action can really support your exhibition of an assignment. So hopefully, if you dress like a tennis ace, you'll play like one, as well.

Cool off

Sundays usually are rest days for Swan, yet if you happen to discover her in the exercise center that day, it's not because she's working out seven days per week. "I give my body a full day's rest regardless." Truly, it's the best time for your muscles to recuperate, and it's so significant for your muscles to have the option to develop, yet a full day's rest is going to rest your mind, as well. Permit yourself to decompress.

Put rest days in your calendar similarly as you would workouts to keep away from abuse wounds and abundant time for muscle fix. Furthermore, recall a good rest intellectually and truly sets you up to carry your A-game to the following workout.

Change your mind

There is nothing of the sort as a convenient solution for your wellbeing and fitness goals, and accept the initial step begins inside you. "It's not just about working out. It's tied in with working within."

The fitness reasoning by which she lives and instructs includes this hypothesis: "Change your mindset to change your life!" You'll frequently hear her shouting to a pressed turn studio. "You need to move toward fitness and life from a solid, positive, tenacious spot. Be fearless in all that you do."

Eat Often

You loathe being furious the same amount as your companions hate to associate with somebody who's bad-tempered from a thundering stomach and low glucose. Stay away from that feeling, and make sure you have the energy needed to take on your next workout by eating for the duration of the day. The key is to think little, fulfilling snacks, not full, heavy meals.

Set achievable goals

Setting a very grandiose, ridiculous, or undesirable goal is simply setting yourself up for disappointment or depletion. "If you don't make the advancement you need to find, for the time being, you could state 'goodness this doesn't work, so I just won't do it,'" she cautions.

The key thing for her to recall and what she tells customers is that consistency and life span are a higher priority than an approaching right-now goal. "My goal is to carry on with a sound lifestyle, and to be a functioning human," she says. "Resting for a day or taking a stroll, over the long haul, doesn't make a difference. There's such a great amount of space for breaks."

Snatch a pen

A diary is a spot for you to hold your abrupt motivations. "I think of expressions or mantras that fly into my mind and record them or make a [digital] banner to impart to my adherents on the web—feeling unmotivated? Think about every one of those positive vibes you composed previously."

You may realize that food journaling or recording your food admission for the day, can assist you with getting thinner. In any case, did you recognize normally writing down your feelings could effectively affect your mind also? Journaling has been appeared to help oversee tension, reduce stress, and organize your feelings by going about as a sound outlet to communicate emotions.

Battle weariness

You've most likely heard an educator reveal to you that

if a move or class doesn't challenge you, it doesn't change you. Not exclusively are they referring to the physiological impacts of exercise, but at the same time, they're cautioning you against smugness.

Blend things up to keep away from the regular old daily schedule, or you'll immediately get exhausted and unmotivated. "If I begin to get exhausted, I know something needs to be balanced. I return it to the books, the pictures, and the music because that is the thing that works best for me."

Do what you love

Although I halted officially rehearsing move when I entered adulthood, that enthusiasm for development and action is the thing that at last drove her to seek after a profession in fitness. "It was wellbeing related and kept my portable. I get the opportunity to see different people each day and stay moving. This work makes me better."

Consider a portion of your preferred pastimes or exercises. Even if you don't transform that energy into a vocation, it's essential to keep up your association with what makes the best sound, glad form of you.

CHAPTER SEVENTEEN: EMOTIONAL CONTROL

Emotions are the most present, squeezing, and sometimes difficult power in our lives. We are driven step by step by our emotions. We take risks because we're energized for new possibilities. We cry because we've been harmed, and we make sacrifices because we love. Beyond question, our emotions direct our thoughts, goals, and actions with better authority than our reasonable minds. In any case, when we follow up on our emotions too rapidly, or we follow up on an inappropriate sort of emotions, we frequently make choices that we later mourn.

Our feelings can adjust between perilous boundaries. Veer excessively far to one side, and you're verging on rage. Steer a lot to one side, and you're in a condition of rapture. Likewise, with numerous different parts of life, emotions are best met with a feeling of balance and a consistent point of view. It is not necessarily the case that we should prevent ourselves from beginning to look all starry eyed at or bouncing for bliss after incredible news. These genuinely are the better things in life. It is negative emotions that must be taken care of with extraordinary consideration.

Negative emotions, similar to wrath, jealousy or sharpness, will generally winding wild, particularly following they've been activated. In time, these sorts of emotions can develop like weeds, gradually molding the mind to work on impeding feelings and commanding day by day life. Ever met an individual who's reliably furious or antagonistic? They weren't brought into the world that way. Yet, they permitted certain emotions to mix within them for such a long time that they became ingrained feelings emerging very much of the time.

So how might we abstain from working on an inappropriate sort of feelings and ace our emotions under the harshest of conditions?

Follow my six stages to control your emotions and recapture soundness in any difficult situation:

Try not to respond immediately. Responding quickly to emotional triggers can be a gigantic mix-up. It is ensured that you'll state or accomplish something you'll later lament. Before discrediting the trigger with your emotional contention, take a full breath, and balance out the mind-boggling motivation. Keep on breathing profoundly for five minutes, feeling like your muscles intensely, and your pulse comes back to typical. As you become calmer, avow to yourself, this is just impermanent.

Request divine direction. Confidence is our

redeeming quality in our darkest minutes. Regardless of your statement of faith, developing a sound connection with the awesome world will assist you with overcoming your obstructions more easily. This is because when you put stock in a higher power, you additionally have faith in the intensity of celestial mediation to give you what you should do, show you why something is going on or even spare you from a specific undesirable situation. At the point when troubled with emotion, close your eyes, imagine a positive answer for your concern, and request that the universe light up the best way ahead.

Locate a sound outlet. Since you've dealt with your emotion, you'll need to discharge it in a sound way. Emotions ought to never be restrained. Call or go see somebody you trust and relate to them what occurred. Getting the point of view other than your own expands your mindfulness. Keep a diary and move your emotions from your internal identity onto the paper. Numerous people think that it's accommodating to take part in forceful exercises, for example, kickboxing or hand to hand fighting, to release their feelings. Others believe and serenade to come back to a quiet condition. Play out whatever movement is most appropriate to you to free your being from repressed sentiments.

See the master plan. Each event of our lives, regardless of whether good or bad, fills a more serious need. Knowledge implies having the option to see past the second and recognize the more prominent significance of some random situation. You may not comprehend it to start with; however, as time passes by, you'll begin to see the master plan falling into immaculate request. Even amidst an emotionally upsetting second, believe that there exists an extreme reason which you will come to appreciate soon.

Supplant your thoughts. Negative emotions tie us to repeating negative thoughts, creating patterns of out and out negative examples. At whatever point you are defied with an emotion which is causing you to feel or think something bad, constrain it insane and supplant it with a different thought. Envision the perfect goals to your difficult playing out, consider somebody who makes you cheerful or recall an event that makes you grin.

Pardon your emotional triggers. Your emotional triggers might be your closest companion, your relatives, yourself or the entirety of the above mentioned. You may feel a sudden flood of outrage when your companion "does that thing she does," or a wound of self-hatred when you remember something you could have done any other way. Be that as it may, when you pardon, you disengage. You separate from the hatred, the desire or the wrath waiting within you. You permit people to be who they are without the need for raising emotions. As you excuse, you will wind up disassociating from the unforgiving feelings appended to your being.

1. Catalyst

It might appear to be basic; however, the first, and maybe generally powerful, the aptitude of emotional dominance is the negligible ability to tune into your feelings. You may not even notify the minutes where you select shirking or minimization as opposed to tuning in. Have you at any point had somebody ask a neighborly, "How are you?" that provoked you to react with a natural "Fine," although you knew wholeheartedly that your reaction was an innocent embellishment? How might you be able to conceivably capture this caring individual's time by clarifying a novel of information for how horrible your day has been? These apparently first harmless minutes cause us to make a habit of dominating and detaching from our emotions. Instead, notice when these examples occur. Be prepared to be a pen, wiling, and helpless, as you venture out emotional health by paying attention to your earnest feelings.

2. Rewind

When tuning into your emotions, make a stride or two in reverse. Ask yourself, "How could I arrive?" Hunt for the triggers that may have added to your feelings. Did your companion's remark about your closet strike a more profound harmony than both of you would have anticipated? Is it true that you are genuinely angry at your accomplice asking you, "What's for supper?" or would you say you are just depleted from a difficult day at work? Understanding where our emotions emerge from and what brings out them is a vital part of assisting you with starting to oversee emotions. At the point when you notice your emotions, be eager to chase for the triggers that may have pushed you into your given feelings.

3. Quick Forward

At the point when we become emotionally elevated, a typical and devastating reaction is rumination. Not after a short time, our thoughts circle us, and we become tied up in our own feelings. A tip to emotional administration is to step out of your zone to increase point of view. Move forward from that second and consider what may occur. What are the results of our actions? Is it accurate to say that we are exclusively affected or do our emotional reactions sparkle others' also? In that future-arranged view, consider what makes a difference to you at that time. Having the option to increase our viewpoint and interface with our definitive qualities causes us to adjust our thoughts and feelings when we come back to the current second.

4. Zoom In

Improving emotional insight is incomprehensible without mindfulness. You have discovered that it is fundamental to tune in and to increase an expanded viewpoint, be that as it may, it is additionally key to dive further. Zoom into the second itself. How would you realize you are the feeling the way you trust you are? Is it true that you are signaling into the butterflies in your stomach? Or then again maybe your hustling heart? Although emotions are experienced around the world, the experience of emotions is somewhat abstract. Immersing yourself in the second will help you see your own signs so that you are more likely to adapt to your coping skills.

5. Screen the Volume

What would you be able to hear? Anything? Emotional authority won't be cultivated on quiet, that is without a doubt. In any case, even if you can hear anything what, or whom, would you be able to hear? Is it the voice of your inward pundit causing feelings of distress or the voice of your grandma giving a shout out to you from the sidelines? Tuning in to the voices in our minds can assist us in evaluating our associations between our thoughts and feelings. In social situations, particularly clashes, we frequently communicate our own story stronger than others. Putting ourselves on quiet while we increment the volume of people around us can be a prudent practice in sympathy and can help us in expanding our points of view.

6. Change the Brightness

Negative emotions can weigh intensely on our work. You may see that in the wake of giving one dim feeling access, it might welcome its similarly unwanted and vindictive companions. When somewhat bothered, without checking your emotions, this sentiment can easily develop to the tumult, dissatisfaction, outrage, and even fury. What to do about this unexpected bad group? Positive emotions will, in general, have a comparable habit and can be similarly as incredible. Modify the splendor to focus on invite emotions. Focus on appreciation right now to bring out related feelings of joy and satisfaction.

7. Press Pause

A tip for emotional administration that can be applied in the present is to press the respite button. Short on time? This easily pertinent expertise is expected to take not precisely a moment. This strategy is especially helpful when you check out your emotions expanding.

For instance, if you zoom in and notice your tension developing, press stop on the situation. Two supportive ways to help with keeping up a mindful moment, especially when matched, are (1) profound breathing, and (2) including. Breathing in through your nose tally gradually to five. During this time, focus on the changes in your body as an impact of your breathing; you may see your lungs extend, your shoulders widen, and your midsection may move. Hold for a second and afterward breathe out, tallying in reverse from five, despite everything keeping up focus on your breath as it goes through your body. Even though it is brief, this mindfulness strategy can help you in recapturing your balance while getting emotionally increased.

8. Stop

A moment isn't always adequate to battle our incredible emotions. To prevent your emotions, assuming responsibility for you, you should know your limit. When do you need to step away? If you are engaged with an apparently useless gathering where you end up butting heads with all individuals, would you say you are mindful of what amount struggle you can deal with before you are at your edge?

When stopping and point of view may not be sufficient, it is useful to be proactive in realizing when to stop yourself. A key way to squeeze stop is to expel yourself from the situation, change the earth or switch your focus if conceivable. Is it accurate to say that you are ready to leave the workplace? Take a walk? Have a glass of water? Shifting your focus can enable you to reduce emotional excitement and recover lucidity, working, and profitability.

9. Mood killer

You may end up shackled to your telephone and fastened to your PC. The interconnectivity of our cutting edge world can make us be easily overwhelmed. Discover harmony between screen time and your time. Set aside an effort to disengage from the world and reconnect with your mind, heart, and soul.

Free of distractions, killing the clamor of the world and its commitments permit you to reduce the brown haze that might be obfuscating your emotional mindfulness and the executives. Utilize these minutes to think about situations where you needed to squeeze respite or stop. Returning to these events with a clear mind may help you in framing an improved point of view.

10. Revive

It is undoubtedly gutsy to pick the undertaking of emotional development. You could select the alternative of auto-pilot instead, giving up from the need to utilize the conceivably time-expanding and energy-depleting controls noted previously. You are bold to leave in this way. It's anything but a simple one; however, it will demonstrate beneficial at long last.

To help climate the difficulties along with your excursion, think about this: How would you revive? This inquiry isn't easily replied in a 10-tip article because the technique changes from person to person. For one person, it might be contemplation, and for another, it might be a petition. For one person, it might be a stimulating workout, and for another, it might be investing quality energy with family. In the best case, you will discover different techniques to revive, giving you a few open doors for self-care, restoration, and improving your emotional prosperity.

A steady reminder of our passionate nature, emotions flood through us at each second of the day. Be that as it may, we regularly take wrong actions when wrong feelings channel through our mind without restriction. To evade the consumption of carrying on during an emotional upsurge, find a way to calm your increased soul and calm your uncomfortable mind. At the point when the second has gone (looking back), you'll be thankful you had the option to be the ace of your emotions.

CHAPTER EIGHTEEN: HEALTHY HABITS TO FEEL BETTER

Everybody is attempting to make a superior life for themselves, regardless of whether for work or personal goals, every one of us has a more profound want (possibly more grounded than you understand) to need to achieve something that will make us feel at last fulfilled. Regardless of how we endeavor to achieve those goals, though, there are difficulties that prevent us and make it difficult. It is NEVER a simple street. Also, uneasiness, brutal working conditions, and stress could make you get bad habits that are possible dangers to your prosperity. That is the reason you ought to be searching for good neutralizing habits that can improve your health and fortify your resolve. When you locate the best habits that coordinate your lifestyle, at that point, you are a considerably more strong way to a more joyful and additionally fulfilling life, full of achievements and positive thoughts.

Unexpected weakness and low energy levels can negatively affect all aspects of your life. Your innovative flash can be decimated, leaving you with zero motivation and thoughts. Work would become dull and hard going, and your public activity would turn into a sorry excuse for what it used to be.

Life for you would never again be entertaining. It's a sorry situation.

What you need to change your life is a more beneficial lifestyle. One that will bring back your common energy and pizzazz.

By learning the best healthy habits to take and following the tips in this article, you'll have the option to return to this ideal state.

What makes a healthy habit?

You might be amazed to discover that more than 40 percent of the actions you play out each day aren't really chosen by you. They're really habits. Habits direct how we live, how we perform, and the outcomes we achieve in life. This is the reason it is so essential to have solid, positive habits.

If you're considering what habits comprise of, consider them along these lines: something that you consistently manage without having to consider intentionally.

"As per the Medical Dictionary, a healthy habit is a conduct that is useful to one's physical or emotional well-being, frequently connected to a significant level of order and poise."

Positive habits are the premise of your success, while

healthy habits improve your general prosperity and make you feel good. Good habits incorporate things like ordinary exercise, a decent eating routine, promptness, keeping guarantees, and so on.

Positive habits make it feasible for us to get things done without burning through extreme mental energy. For example, rather than intuition how to stroll down the steps in a morning, this is dealt with by your inner mind, which has taken in the habit of walking securely down steps. You don't need to consider moving your legs, and controlling your equalization, and so forth.

Healthy habits to improve each part of your life

Presently you comprehend what habits are and the advantages positive habits offer, how about we investigate now at these healthy habits you ought to embrace to change your life. These habits are broken into four areas:

- Healthy eating habits
- Healthy living habit
- Healthy habits for a tranquil mind
- Healthy relationship habits

1. Make sure you bite your food well

The vast majority eat down their food and don't set aside the effort to bite or appreciate it appropriately. If you're one of these people, take a stab at hindering your eating by biting your food longer than you would regularly do. You'll appreciate the flavor of your food more, and you're probably going to eat less as well.

2. Stock up on healthy food

At home, you nibble on what's in your pantries, more relaxed, and freezer. If all you have in there is ultra-prepared foods like fries, chocolate, and frozen yogurt, at that point, you'll wind up nibbling on them (not a pleasant thought). To get out from under this habit, make sure you have heaps of healthy foods in your home like dried organic products, seeds, and nuts to help fulfill your appetite yearnings.

3. Expect to complete 10,000 stages every day

Sounds like a great deal? It's really the base sum suggest by fitness specialists. It's not very difficult to arrive at 10,000 stages in a day. Basically, stroll in the recreation center toward the beginning of the day and evening, and use the stairwell rather than the lift at work.

4. Go for a stroll at lunchtime

Lunchtimes don't need to be only for eating. You can utilize the time to get some important air, light, and exercise. I usually stroll for half of my mid-day break – the other half I leave for eating.

5. Freeze your foods grown from the ground

This is an extraordinary thing to do, as freezing these

foods implies they'll go on until you're prepared to eat them. What's more, obviously you can freeze them when they're at their pinnacle, so they'll taste extraordinary when defrosted and additionally cooked. This method is additionally an eminent way to appreciate healthy products of the soil outside of their typical occasional accessibility.

6. Focus on hues, not calories

Such a large number of people put their well-being and diet focus on what number of calories they are expending each day. In any case, a healthy eating routine isn't just about calories.

For instance, there is a major difference between eating a bunch of raw nuts and a similar calorie measure of cake. Without a doubt, the last may taste better to you – however, the nuts will always be the more beneficial decision.

7. Include an extra serving of greens to your plate

One basic way to help your intake of healthy foods is to include an extra serving of greens to every one of your meals. If you ordinarily eat a hamburger and French fries (not suggested!), begin including a part of peas or a green serving of mixed greens to your plate. After some time, you can start expanding the greens – and diminishing the shoddy nourishment.

8. Be dynamic outside the exercise center

I'm sure you've spotted people at work who go to the exercise center most morning. They surely realize how to begin their day well; however, watch their habits after that. Frequently they plunk during unsurpassed at their work area, and no uncertainty return home and relax before the TV.

While setting off to the rec center is excellent, don't make it your most important thing in the world. Get out in the outside air and regular light and move your body the way nature planned – by strolling and running.

9. Eat carbs consistently

Every now and then, carbs leave style. We're cautioned their bad for us, and we ought to dodge them. In any case, no-carb and low-carb consume fewer calories, for the most part, end up as trends. That is because carbs are really are a superb wellspring of energy for our bodies.

Our predecessors lived and flourished with carb-heavy weight control plans for a great many years. Simply make sure you're picking healthy carbs rather than refined carbs.

10. Pick healthy fats

Not all fats are the equivalent. Some are good for us; some are definitely not. Which are the healthy fats? If you stick to cold-squeezed extra-virgin olive oil, nuts, and avocados, you'll be getting the basic supplements you need – in the most beneficial structures accessible.

11. Try not to eat until you're full

A healthy person's stomach is the size of a clench hand, while an unhealthy person's stomach can be the size of a football. It's a stunning reality. The reason for the twisted stomach extension is overeating. At the point when this is done routinely, the stomach begins to extend. Thus, the person needs to eat increasingly more to keep up that full, fulfilled feeling.

How to stay away from this? Always eat somewhat less than you might suspect you need or might want. This will keep your stomach at its characteristic size – and your body at a healthy weight as well.

12. Cut down on your meat intake

Have you known about meat-free Mondays? This is actually as it sounds, don't eat meat every Monday. If you're a major meat eater, at that point, meat-free Mondays are an extraordinary way to promptly reduce your meat intake. What's more, it will likewise acquaint you with the tasty flavors accessible in a veggie lover and vegetarian meals.

13. Divide your sugar intake

We as a whole realize that sugar is bad for us, however yet, a large portion of us, despite everything, expend masses of it every day. The issue obviously is that sugar tastes extraordinary. So good, truth be told, that we truly become dependent on it.

Presently, if I instructed you to go 'without any weaning period' and cut out sugar entirely from your eating routine tomorrow – you will most likely not have the option to do so. That is the reason I suggest a sensible and achievable goal of splitting your sugar intake. You can do this through simple advances like lessening or removing sugar in tea or espresso, halting adding sugar to your grains, and picking healthier tidbits.

14. Trade soft drinks for water

Soft drinks are regularly full of sugar (or artificial sugars), shading, and different nasties! They may taste good; however, they'll leave you feeling bad. Instead, dump the soft drinks and change to drinking mineral water or separated faucet water. Your body will much be obliged.

15. Purchase a reusable water jug and keep it around your work area

I used to come into the workplace and drink tea or espresso throughout the day. I never thought about drinking water. At that point, I began to see that a few people acquired huge, reusable water bottles that they continued tasting from all through the working day. I chose to give this a go, and I was astounded by the fact that it was so natural to drink in an abundance of 500ml of water each day. Furthermore, the best thing? I saw

that I felt increasingly hydrated, progressively focused –
and certainly healthier in general. Attempt it for
yourself, and I'm sure, similar to me, you'll never come
to work without your water bottle.

16. Quit gauging yourself

This connects to my prior remarks about calories. A few
people – maybe including yourself – are focused on
their weight. They gauge themselves each morning and
consistently. If they lose weight, they're blissful. Be that
as it may, if they put on weight, they can rapidly give in
to wretchedness.

Presently, kindly don't misunderstand me, you
positively ought to mean to have a healthy weight. In
any case, this will be a characteristic outcome of eating
healthily and practicing regularly.

17. Pick charming exercise

You may be putting off practicing as you don't care for
setting off to the rec center or running neglected
climate. Rather, why not pick fun exercises like moving,
yoga or group activity? At the point when exercise is fun,
you'll have considerably more motivation to do it
regularly.

18. Stay away from overworking out

People who over-exercise will generally age speedier
than they should. Most things in life come down to
adjust, and exercise is no exemption. Over practicing for

quite a long time and years will exhaust your body of its vital energy – leaving you emptied and feeling from sync.

19. Hit the sack 30 minutes sooner than expected

In today's age of Netflix and YouTube, it's very simple to wind up, observing only one more video. Pre-web, you'd have likely hit the sack a few hours sooner than you at present do. My recommendation? You have a caution to get you up in the first part of the day. What about setting an alert to notify you when it's time to kill the TV and get yourself to bed.

20. Mood killer innovation every once in a while

Innovation is an extraordinary thing. It empowers me to type these words – and for you to understand them. Be that as it may, let's face it, it's very simple to get dependent on our TVs, PCs, tablets, and cell phones. Most of the people are gazing at one of these gadgets for the vast majority of their morning, evening, evening, and past. It's a constant universe of messages, SMS messages, news channels, online networking refreshes, and so on.

My recommendation? Make sure you step out of this pattern of distraction by having regular breaks from your gadgets. For instance, why not switch off the entirety of your gadgets when you're eating with your friends and family? Make discussion be your focus, rather than being consumed by online stuff.

Healthy habits for a quiet mind

21. Invest energy in nature

Being outside has been found to profoundly affect your mental wellbeing chiefly because of the introduction to daylight expanding your serotonin levels. Exploration has likewise discovered that spending even a short measure of time around nature helps your state of mind. Envision going through a day in a spot this way:

22. Have something to anticipate

Being in a condition of positive expectation and hope can expand your bliss level. Planning something you appreciate and relax because of, regardless of whether it's an excursion, an arranged run, getting friends or twisting together with that book you've always needed to peruse can shield you from harping on any negatives.

23. Reflect

Meditation is presumably the most discussed idea in the bliss camps, and it has good motivations to be interchangeable with good mental health. Studies have shown regular meditation rehearses reduce stress, uneasiness, and health issues. The principal reason is it can help reduce overthinking and make an increasingly mindful mindset. It can come as simply sitting unobtrusively, yoga, supplication or intentional breathing.

24. Move your body

Endorphins are the synthetic concoctions in the cerebrum that essentially reduce the view of agony. At the point when you move your bodies, these are discharged and basically tell your cerebrum that everything is great. Even if it's simply getting up from your seat, moving around while doing the housework, or taking up a regular exercise schedule, these actions can build the feel-good synthetic compounds and lift your state of mind.

25. Gain some new useful knowledge

People who keep on learning into adulthood have more noteworthy by and large wellbeing. This could be because the cerebrum is continually being revived and overhauled yet, also the sense of achievement, good faith, and distraction it makes. As it were, it gives you reason and focuses on expanding the capacity to adapt to stress. So get familiar with another language, take up painting or join up with a course you've always liked doing to make increasingly mental wellbeing.

26. Accomplish something decent for someone

Graciousness might be viewed as simply good habits, yet being genuinely kind towards others builds your satisfaction just like theirs. Positive social interactions, regardless of how little they may appear, helps your feel-good vibrations. Offering praises with unadulterated goals, holding an entryway open, or offering to pay for a more bizarre's espresso will keep you feeling suitable for the remainder of the day. Do this regularly, and you'll keep your positive mindset bested up just as creating satisfaction for someone else.

27. Reexamine harmful relationships

Sometimes people's mental wellbeing decreases because they become acclimated to being around people who cut them down. This can damage their self-regard and self-worth; however, they frequently don't connect this with others. You are the whole of the five people you're around the most. Ask yourself, are these five people supportive, kind, and amusing to be near? If not, it might be time to reexamine your relationships.

28. Detox carefully

The risks of an excessive amount of internet-based life are regularly said. The correlation game can make you feel emptied and like disappointments if we're not living how others are at present living. This in itself is motivation to have a time of detox from your telephone or PC. The advanced world, as much as possible, remove our current moments and permits us to miss what's truly going on around us. Detoxing will give you that sense of freedom of time to do different things that will help your mental health.

29. Rest more

Rest regularly gets overlooked when we're living occupied lives; however, that is no reason. Getting sufficient rest is vital to an ideal healthy mind. Lack of sleep causes temperament swings, fractiousness, health issues, and all-round dysfunction that affects how we think and makes us respond negatively to things occurring in our day by day lives. More rest likens to a sense of harmony and motivation during your time rather than stress and uneasiness.

30. Get things done without anyone else

Low self-worth or self-regard can make people accept that they can't get things done without anyone else. The need to always have someone to get things done with can make a sense of neediness and absence of self-love. Going off and getting things done without anyone else manufactures certainty and a sense of freedom.

Try not to be reluctant to be distant from everyone else and make time for yourself; it's a great way to consider yourself and have a breather away from others indeed.

31. Offer thanks

Appreciation has been found to expand bliss and reduce stress creating a progressively positive mindset. People frequently get made up for lost time with what turned out poorly in their day, even if most of what happened was positive. A good habit to begin is to thoroughly consider your day and note everything that was incredible – from the straight-forward drive to work, a grin from an outsider, the tasty food you had for lunch, or a book from your friend.

32. Sit and stand upright

Body language is firmly associated with our mindset. At the point when you slump, it subconsciously makes the general feeling of threatening vibe, languor, and antagonism. At the point when we sit or stand upright, it makes the feeling of power and certainty.

33. Discover something to chuckle about

Chuckling is powerful as it reduces stress levels, improves mindset, and even momentary memory. Chuckling along with someone is most likely the best sort of giggling, but simply viewing an entertaining TV show or even snickering without anyone else can work.

34. Record things

Recording things is extremely powerful because, in the demonstration of composing, the cerebrum forms what's being recorded more gradually; thus, it turns into a sort of treatment. It can assist you with handling emotions and identify difficult regions or constraining convictions that ceaseless overthinking makes more regrettable. Recording goals and dreams can realize a positive lift, and making arrangements of past achievements can help show you the successes in your life.

35. Invest energy with your pet

Any caring creature can build your feelings of energy in little and significant ways. They decline dejection, get you dynamic, make cherishing bonds, keep you present at the time and give you reason.

36. Change your everyday practice

While routine can keep us comfortable, it likewise makes sense of everyday life and can bring about misery. Rolling out simply little improvements in your routine can fool the mind into believing you're accomplishing something completely different. It could be taking a different course to work, strolling as opposed to taking the transport, heading off to someplace different for lunch or getting up somewhat prior toward the beginning of the day. Switching things up makes assortment and frees you up to different encounters and opportunities.

37. Investigate your city or town

Being a traveler in your own town or city isn't something people will generally consider. Imagine you're visiting just because – what neighborhoods would you visit? Where might you eat? Doing this can enable you to acknowledge where you live and increase a different perspective to a recognizable spot, which assists open with increasing the mind.

38. Practice absolution

Absolution can be a hard idea for some. In any case, a

great deal of our apprehension is brought about by our powerlessness to release things and proceed onward. This doesn't mean approving what someone has done, but simply dropping the cynicism around it and pushing ahead. Studies have shown that absolution ensures against stress, and excusing yourself is important excessively to discharge any baggage and self-detest and make a happy life.

39. Associate with someone

As social creatures, we blossom with the association. At the point when you're feeling discouraged, the exact opposite thing you need to do is a discussion or contact others. Remember that conversing with people, even simply short discussions with friends or in support groups, can fix your sense of disengagement gigantically. Relationships with others manufacture a sense of having a place and self-worth, so make time to associate with someone.

40. Go through a day being mindful

This is an incredible way to look at how you travel as the day progressed. How does your morning meal taste? How do your legs feel when you're strolling? Where did the elements for your lunch originate from? What emotions would you say you are feeling in every moment?

Try not to pass judgment on yourself yet simply be in every moment. Carrying your mind to the current moment can help reduce wretchedness all the while.

41. Think about a progressively positive perspective

A negative mindset makes a negative life. If you're in this class of considering them to be as always being half vacant, possibly question why you think along these lines. It could basically come from convictions you've gotten; however, comprehend there is always a decision by the way you see things.

Decide to consider a different, progressively positive perspective next time. Doing this regularly will gradually help change the way you take a gander at your general surroundings.

42. Quit taking photographs of everything

While it's extraordinary to take photographs for tokens, investing an excess of energy snapping the picture as opposed to getting a charge out of the moment can diminish our satisfaction. Therapist Maryanne Garry of the Victoria University of Wellington in New Zeal has discovered taking unending photographs "controls both our recollections and emotional translations of lived experiences," meaning we wind up recalling less and don't fully value the moment.

43. Grin (even if it's phony)

Certifiable grins portray our cheerful internal feelings; however, research has found even phony grinning fools the mind into believing we're happy. So also if you're in a peaceful room without anyone else, grin and you'll see overtime, it makes sense of mental wellbeing.

44. Accomplish something that is out of your usual range of familiarity

One of the primary reasons people can become discouraged is their need to stay comfortable. Accuse this for the cerebrum; it's doing everything it can to prevent you from accomplishing something frightful because it's an endurance system – if you're comfortable at that point you're sheltered.

Breaking out of safe places is never as frightening as your cerebrum envisions it to be, and it makes certainty, wellbeing and opens up new and energizing possibilities. The outcome? Better mental health.

Healthy relationship habits

45. Regard your loved ones

The establishment of any good relationship is the degree of regard within it. Being straightforward, maintaining a strategic distance from tattle, and esteeming your loved ones for the exceptional people, they are establishing the pace for every one of your interactions.

46. Express gratitude toward them

Showing appreciation can be as simple as a verbal "thank you" or a short note, yet the impacts are expansive. Regardless of whether your partner simply did a heap of dishes or your friend plunged in at the eleventh hour to make all the difference, don't pass up on the opportunity to express profound gratitude.

47. Communicate

If you truly love someone, don't be hesitant to tell them. State, "I love you," frequently, and when you state it, don't joke about this. Tell your significant other, friends, and family the amount you care about them. Be liberal with your affection.

48. Go for a stroll

Going for a walk through the area is an incredible way to reconnect with your friend or partner. These strolls are an incredible opportunity to get some outside air and get up to speed with life without spending an exorbitant price.

49. Make each other chuckle

Cleverness is a powerful way to bond with each other. Never pass up on an opportunity to make your loved ones giggle. Be a numskull, watch a satire, and don't be reluctant to split a joke at your own cost periodically.

50. Set goals together

This habit is particularly important for romantic relationships, in which you're working as a group. At the point when you don't set goals together, you hazard subverting each other. Joining to defeat a test is a powerful way to bond.

51. Take up another pastime

Nothing executes friendships and sentiments quicker than fatigue. Try not to allow things to deteriorate. Get another leisure activity that you're both inspired by once in a while. Challenge each other to consummate your aptitudes, and receive the rewards of becoming together.

52. Accomplish something decent "because"

Extraordinary amazement requires thoughtfulness. It very well may be as simple as showing up with some espresso or getting your partner's preferred treat on your way home. Send your mom a bunch of roses aimlessly, or offer to assist your friend with a task. You'll make their day and show them the amount you give it a second thought.

53. Loosen up together

It's not essential to transform each moment together into a detailed excursion. Friendships and romantic relationships with staying power are those who can flourish in everyday situations. Figure out how to love sitting in front of the TV together, taking strolls, or sharing simple meals.

54. Set aside effort for yourselves

Even the closest couples and friends need time to investigate their individual advantages. You don't need to like very similar things to get along. Your independence is likely a piece of what attracted you to each other. Make sure that you and your loved ones get time to sustain their gifts and interests.

55. Reconnect regularly

Messaging and calling day in and day out is certifiably not a healthy habit, yet getting in contact is incredible for a romantic relationship. For friends and family, it isn't important to communicate something specific consistently, yet interfacing occasionally allows you to share your lives.

56. Do tasks together

For couples, working in the house together prevents one gathering from feeling angry toward the other. A recent report found that 62% of couples accept that sharing errands prompts a successful partnership.

57. Set aside some effort to cuddle

Physical contact impacts how you feel about your significant other. The demonstration of snuggling makes your bodies discharge oxytocin, a hormone liable for holding. Embracing additionally causes the arrival of oxytocin, so this healthy habit applies to non-romantic relationships also.

58. Mention to them what you love about them

Saying, "I love you," is extraordinary, but sometimes it's

ideal to back up the sentiment up with certain models. Tell your friends and partner what specific qualities you love about them. This certainty support causes them to face whatever hardships come their way.

59. Pay attention

Posing thoughtful inquiries and reacting may appear presence of mind, but numerous friends, family, and love relationships need mindfulness. Listen profoundly. Make eye to eye connection. At the point when a loved one converses with you, they should feel that they have your full focus.

60. Make sense of their love language (and talk it)

Insider facts to Love that Last reveals to us that there are five fundamental ways that people give and get love. Knowing your significant other's love language causes you to gain proficiency with the ideal ways to show your passion dependent on their needs. It's important that love languages are not restricted to romantic relationships.

61. Get some information about their day

This is an extraordinary way to begin any discussion, regardless of whether your visitation to your father or conversing with your closest friend. You'll get a huge amount of data that can assist you with being available for them, and you'll show that you're genuinely intrigued by their life by posing this simple inquiry.

62. Be straightforward

Trustworthiness is basic for any relationship. At the point when you care about someone long, you should have the option to come clean with them. They depend on you to be someone they can trust. Besides, it's kinder than lying, and you never need to stress over them, discovering that you lied.

63. Be their cheerleader

We all experience difficulties, but having someone who can support you on your most noticeably awful day is a genuine gift. Be the person who can give them the encouragement they need to confront whatever is before them. Sometimes your loved ones simply need to realize that you put stock in them.

64. Unplug to reconnect

You can't have quality time if you have your heads covered in your telephones, computer games, or PCs. You can positively appreciate those things with each other, yet focus on hobnobbing screen-free too.

If you're out somewhere else, make a no-screen strategy with the goal that you can effectively hear one out another.

65. Show that you're steadfast

Constancy is an easy decision in a romantic relationship. Devotion isn't the best way to show dependability, though. In the entirety of your relationships, make sure to close down tattle, and defend loved ones even if they can't go to bat for themselves.

66. Be the person they can depend on

Your partner and friends should realize that whether they had a bad day at work, or they're debilitated, you are always prepared to hop in and help. At the point when things are going ineffectively for your family, your folks and kin, realize they can go to you. You're there on time, each time they need you to be, and you mean what you state.

67. Do your fair share

It's out of line to anticipate that one partner or friend should bear the weight for everything. You don't need to divide each duty into halves; however, you do need to agree with the goal that neither of you conveys the heap alone. This applies to things like family unit errands, yet it additionally identifies with things like choosing where to eat or picking an excursion.

68. Make time for them

"The key isn't to organize what's on your calendar, but to plan your needs."

If you need your relationships to last, you need to make them a need. Calendar "arrangements" with loved ones if you experience difficulty making the time to associate with them.

69. Love without judgment

Unless their conduct is a major issue, re-outline how you consider the other person's blemishes. To have genuine love, you need to love the genuine person. To see who someone really is, they need to feel suffciently safe to show you without feeling judged. Your family, friends, and significant others should realize that you love them, imperfections and everything.

70. Excuse their errors

You aren't great, nor are your friends, your partner, or your family. At the point when someone you love fails, come at the situation from their perspective. If it's not worth cutting off the association over the slip-up, pardon the person.

71. Be powerless and acknowledge powerlessness

Being powerless can require practice in friendships and romantic relationships. With friends, this is your opportunity to show them what your identity is, and it allows them to be progressively open with you. With your partner, helplessness with each other forms the trust.

72. Start the day with them

For couples, starting every day with your partner is a show of solidarity. Even if you work inverse calendars, you can discover ways to share the start of another day together. Compose a note or put in almost no time toward the beginning of the day seeing them off.

73. Consider it a day together

You don't really need to be on a similar rest plan as your partner, but slowing down together is a healthy habit. This demonstration constructs trust, and it gives you one progressively opportunity to ponder the day.

74. Make choices as a group

Autonomy is extraordinary; however, when a choice you need to make will seriously affect your family, friends, or partner, it's ideal to remember them for the procedure. Recollect that you're in it together, and set aside an effort to set up how your group will convey about important life choices.

CHAPTER NINETEEN: LOVE YOUR BODY AND YOUR SPIRIT

Saying "thank you" to others is something you learn at an early age. Be that as it may, how regularly do you express gratitude toward yourself?

Saying "thank you" to your body is one of the most important things you can do, particularly when you're seeking a life of self-love and health. It is anything but a habit that quickly falls into place because society is continually advising us to change ourselves to fit a socially accepted standard.

I've committed my life to help change society's desires and make self-love and body acknowledgment a standard idea.

Here are ways you can value your body with simple rituals for self-love and health.

1. Meditation

Meditation is a beautiful way to focus on yourself. At the point when life is stressful, or your mind is hustling, you can always go to meditation. It's additionally open to everybody because you can do it anyplace. You should simply locate a peaceful, comfortable space, close your eyes, and just relax.

At the point when you commit yourself to facilitate your mind each day, you will receive the rewards of meditation as your own health advocate.

2. Mindful development

Moving your body in a mindful way is entirely different than practicing or working out. This isn't tied in with constraining yourself to accomplish something you despise. This is tied in with checking out your body and asking yourself what you need. One of my preferred ways to move my body is strolling outside with my pooches. I take a gander at the sky, the blossoms, the trees, and the magnificence surrounding me. I become present and mindful. I love the way my body feels.

Figure out how to move that makes both your body and mind feel good. Possibly a climb or a yoga class is what you're searching for? If you haven't discovered your mindful development of decision, continue looking. Because the best part about discovering it is that you get the chance to pick something you appreciate!

3. A good read

At the point when I initially began investigating self-love, I honestly didn't have the foggiest idea what it implied. I realized how to love someone else, yet how the hell do I love myself? My personal self-love venture eventually started at a yoga class.

Finding a book (or books!) that addresses you is a critical part of self-love and wellbeing for the mind. Lose yourself in a book shop. Stroll through the self-love book passageway and see what picks you.

4. Encircle yourself with bliss

Where do you invest the majority of your energy? Is it your work area at work? Is it your vehicle? When you check out your environmental factors, do you feel an eruption of delight? If not, the subsequent stage is to make a domain you love entirely.

My preferred things to encircle myself with are new blossoms, positive messages, pictures of people I love, salt lights, basic oils, and my preferred books. It's a demonstration of self-love when you are in a comfortable situation full of the things that bring you bliss. At the point when you can grin by merely glancing around, you're rehearsing self-love!

5. Request help

Self-love is requesting help. At the point when you're making some hard memories, you'll be astonished that the vast majority would like to be there for you. It might be difficult to be powerless and request help, but perhaps the ideal ways to overcome an extreme time is getting the support you need.

It's alright not to be alright. The fact of the matter is, you don't need to experience only it. Requesting the support you need is a gift that you get the opportunity to give yourself.

6. Discover your place of euphoria

We should all have that one spot we can go to and feel happy. For instance, when I need a shot in the arm or a place to restore my spirit, I head to a bistro. Something about taking a seat at a table, encompassed by the positive energy, working on my PC, and tasting on a latte fills my needs.

Consider where you love to go. Is it a stroll along the seashore? A joint with friends? A workout class? An artistry class? Self-love is tied in with topping off your own cup. At the point when your cup is full, you can more readily serve others.

7. Slow down

We live in such a quick-paced condition. Allow yourself to back off, appreciate the remarkable moments, and deal with yourself. Here are a couple of different ways to back off in your day by day life.

Eat gradually. Each time you eat, make it a point to plunk down without distractions. Make sure you bite gradually and really taste what you are eating. This simple practice is a distinct advantage by the way you feel in your body each day.

Relax. During your day, take a few minutes to relax simply. Take ten full breaths and check in with your body. Permit yourself to refocus and refocus before you proceed onward with your day by day undertakings.

Rest. If you can tell that your body or your mind is excessively depleted, you must permit yourself to give your body what it needs. It can be a negative encounter for some because of the unpleasant inward exchange you hear. Try not to tune in to those words. Rather, when you look in the mirror, look at yourself without flinching and state, "I love you." Do it, even if you feel senseless!

Self-talk is demonstrated to work. You can likewise set up a couple of notes on your mirror with positive, cherishing reminders. Awakening each day with a sort and cherishing message to yourself and your body will change the relationship you have with yourself in the best way.

8. Appreciation

Having a morning and nighttime schedule that is devoted to appreciation is a stunning way to support your self-love. And all you need is a diary to begin.

At the point when you get up each morning, and every previous night you rest, record three things for which you're appreciative. It's a beautiful way to respect yourself and your life. It's an ideal time to state thank you to your body!

Takeaway

Keep in mind, self-love is a multifaceted idea. Like some other relationship in your life, the one you have with yourself requires sustaining, persistence, and thoughtfulness. There are numerous ways to rehearse self-love, and these are only a couple. Investigate different strategies for thinking about yourself, and find what makes you feel euphoric and healthy — in your mind, body, and soul.

CHAPTER TWENTY: THE POWER OF REHASHED WORDS AND THOUGHTS

Believing is normally a blend of words, sentences, mental images, and sensations. Thoughts are guests who visit the focal station of the mind. They come, stay some time, and afterward vanish, making space for different thoughts. A portion of these thoughts stay longer, gain power, and affect the life of the person thinking them.

Do you, as the vast majority, let thoughts associated with stresses, fears, outrage or misery consume your mind more often than not?

Do you continue consuming your mind with an inward discussion about negative situations and actions?

Such inward discussion eventually affects the subconscious mind, which acknowledges them as genuine.

It is of vital importance to be cautious about what goes into the subconscious mind. Words and thoughts that are rehashed regularly get more grounded by the reiterations, sink into the subconscious mind and affect the conduct, actions, and reactions of the person in question.

The subconscious mind respects the words and thoughts that get stopped inside it as communicating and portraying a genuine situation, and this way tries to adjust the words and thoughts to the real world. It works perseveringly to make these words and thoughts a reality in the life of the person saying or thinking them.

This implies if you frequently disclose to yourself that it is confusing or challenging to get cash, the subconscious mind will acknowledge your words and put obstructions in your way. If you continue disclosing to yourself that you are rich, it will discover ways to carry you opportunities to get rich and push you towards making the most of these opportunities.

The thoughts that you express through your words shape your life. This is frequently done unconsciously, as barely any pay attention to their thoughts and the words they use while thinking, and let outside conditions and situations figure out what they think about. For this situation, there is no freedom. Here, the outside world affects the inner world.

If you consciously pick the thoughts, expressions, and words that you rehash in your mind, your life will begin to change. You will start creating new situations and conditions. You will utilize the power of affirmations.

Affirmations are sentences that are rehashed regularly during the day and which sink into the subconscious mind, along these lines discharging its huge power to appear the aim of the words and expressions in the outside world. This doesn't imply that each word you articulate will bring results. To trigger the subconscious mind without hesitation, the words must be said with attention, goal and feeling.

To get positive outcomes, affirmations must be expressed in positive words. Take a gander at the accompanying two sentences:

1. I am not feeble any longer.

2. I am trustworthy and authoritative.

Though the two sentences appear to communicate a similar thought, however, in different words, the first is a negative sentence. It makes in the mind a mental image of shortcoming. This isn't the right wording. The subsequent sentence stirs in the mind a mental picture of solidarity.

It isn't sufficient to state an affirmation a couple of times, and afterward anticipate that your life should change. More than this is vital. It is important to certify with attention, just as with powerful urge, confidence and constancy. It is additionally important to pick the right affirmation for a specific situation. You need to feel comfortable with it; in any case, the affirmation may not work or may bring you something that you don't generally need.

Affirmations can be utilized along with creative visualization to fortify it, and they can be used independently, all alone. They are of exceptional importance for people who think that it's difficult to picture. For this situation, they fill in as a replacement for creative visualization.

Rather than repeating negative and pointless words and expressions in the mind, why not pick positive words and expressions to assist you with building the life you need? By selecting your thoughts and words, you exercise control over your life.

Here are some affirmations:

- Step by step, I am turning out to be more joyful and progressively fulfilled.
- With each inward breath, I am filling myself with bliss.
- Love is filling my life now.
- The power of the Cosmos is filling my life with love.
- A ton of cash is streaming now into my life.
- The power of the Universal Mind is currently furnishing my life with riches.
- The powerful and vital energy of the Cosmos is streaming and filling my body and mind.
- Healing energy is continually filling each cell of my body.

- I always stay calm and in control of myself in each situation, and all conditions.
- I am having a brilliant, upbeat, and entrancing day.

CHAPTER TWENTY ONE: AFFIRMATIONS AND THE SUBCONSCIOUS MIND

The power of your subconscious mind goes farther than you may suspect.

No joke proposed.

I'm sure you'll concur with me when I state our minds are very entangled.

Be that as it may, you may be astonished by how much control we have over its programming.

The capacity of your subconscious mind is to store and recover information. Its main responsibility is to guarantee that you react precisely the way you are programmed. Your subconscious mind makes everything you state and do fit an example predictable with your self-idea, your "lord program." This is the reason repeating positive affirmations are so compelling — you can really reprogram your own thought designs by slipping in positive and success-arranged sound chomps.

This is the reason motivational exercises, for example,

perusing rousing statements, are so significant for people committed to positive reasoning. By focusing your thoughts on uplifting thoughts, your subconscious will start to execute a positive example in your way of reasoning and your point of view.

Your subconscious mind is abstract. It doesn't think or reason autonomously; it only complies with the orders it gets from your conscious mind. Similarly, as your conscious mind can be thought of as the plant specialist, planting seeds, your subconscious mind can be thought of as the nursery, or ripe soil, in which the seeds sprout and develop. This is another motivation behind why outfitting the power of positive reasoning is important to the establishment of your whole thought process.

Did you realize that your subconscious mind makes up around 90% of your absolute mind power?

Instead of the conscious mind (which is liable for your everyday exercises when you're alert), which makes up simply 10%?

This is the reason numerous people that attempt to lose weight quit smoking or embrace another habit, neglect to succeed - because they don't realize that the key to success is to get to the subconscious mind and reprogram it with new and empowering data.

Things being what they are, how would you access and change your subconscious mind?

One way is to utilize affirmations. Through reiteration, affirmations strengthen an aim so profoundly that it sidesteps your conscious mind and goes straight into your subconscious.

At the point when this occurs, you begin to encounter change and appreciate the advantages of arriving at your ideal result.

You go from imagining positive intuition to living in constant happiness and appreciation.

Furthermore, this is actually what I need for you!

If you've been battling to expel a negative habit from your day by day schedule and you'd prefer to make the things you genuinely need in life at that point.

Here are some affirmations to reprogram your subconscious mind and lift your mind power today:

My thoughts are leveled out.

The entirety of my thoughts is positive and empowering.

I am full of empowering thoughts from the moment I wake up.

I am profoundly associated with my higher self.

I am an open channel for unending imagination and intelligence.

I trust I can do anything!

Every day I'm developing new and positive habits.

My capacity to vanquish my difficulties is boundless.

My capability to succeed is endless.

I have the power to change my life by changing my thoughts.

By repeating positive affirmations day by day, you are boosting your self-regard and improving your certainty. The most important piece of affirmations is to state/keep in touch with them in the current state, as though it's as of now evident. In doing as such, you are telling your mind this is occurring; that you are as of now this person, and you have the things you need.

Another important piece of affirmations is to feel the emotions that accompany this genuinely. You may begin by setting your hand over your heart as you discuss these mantras. Saying these toward the beginning of the day is an extraordinary way to launch your day!

Also, you know what's even progressively powerful?

At the point when you join the power of affirmations with personal development devices to amplify your manifestations! Because then you have two apparatuses working to reprogram your subconscious mind simultaneously!

CHAPTER TWENTY-TWO: GASTRIC BAND HYPNOSIS (PLACING)

Strategy

Patient position and trocar arrangement. A five-port procedure is utilized, with four 5mm ports and one 15mm port. The patient is put in recumbent with the arms reached out, in the modified lithotomy position, with the specialist remaining between the patient's legs and all furthest points all around cushioned. An orogastric cylinder is utilized for gastric decompression.

A 5mm optical trocar is utilized to get to the stomach pit in the left subcostal district. The situation of the trocars is as per the following: Trocar 1 is embedded subxiphoid in a mid-epigastric position; trocar 2, utilized for liver retraction, is embedded at the patient's right subcostal edge in the mid-clavicular line; trocars 3 and 4, in a curve stretching out from trocar 2 toward the patient's left; and trocar 5, along the side on the left subcostal edge (Figure 1). The point of liver retraction is to lift the liver away from the gastroesophageal edge and spleen, which permits safe dissection at the edge of His.

Point of His dissection. The omentum covering the edge of His is tenderly cleared to the side to encourage presentation during the production of a little entry point parallel on the left half of the gastroesophageal junction within the gastrophrenic tendon; this little "window" starts the plane of dissection for the retrocardial burrow. Care must be taken to save the gastrophrenic connections to help secure the band and keep up the dependability of the fundus. Fat cushions encompassing the gastroesophageal junction can be extracted, if needed, to uncover the stomach divider or identify and fix a crural defect or hiatal hernia.

Standards flaccida dissection. In the lesser omentum ("standards flaccida") dissection at the lesser curvature, the standards flaccida is extended to make an entry point and uncover the right crus. If a huge atypical hepatic supply route exudes from the left gastric vein, the "two-advance" dissection can be utilized by creating an extra perigastric passage over the variant hepatic vessel and close to the lesser curvature.

The purpose of dissection is along the foremost fringe of the right crus, at its most lower perspective. This is the purpose of conjunction of the right and left mainstays of the right crus. The peritoneum is chiseled, and an articulating gruff dissector is presented, embedded at the entry point at the right crus, and tenderly progressed to rise at the edge of His cut. The dissector gets through the right-sided port and passes delicately into this zone of dissection with no torque. It passes an extremely short separation behind the gastroesophageal junction to rise into the effectively dismembered edge of His. This basic advance requires no power by any stretch of the imagination. Any resistance experienced implies that the purpose of dissection at the right crus is excessively high and that the dissector is driving into the throat or stomach or there is a chance of a hiatal hernia with a back sliding segment. For this situation, the dissector ought to be delicately pulled back and embedded caudal to follow another course behind the gastroesophageal junction. Once the dissector gets through the standards flaccida burrow, it is prepared to hold the band by its tubing or stitch circle to get it through.

Hiatal crural fix

The fat cushion around the gastroesophageal junction is evacuated, while "dimpling" of the foremost crus is seen or if there is laxity of the right crus posteriorly. All sliding Hiatal hernias are reduced with the full assembly of the distal throat and fixed principally with back nonabsorbable figure-of-eight stitches. Complete crural introduction posteriorly can be gotten with cautious dissection staying cranial to the lesser sac. If no sliding part is envisioned, however, a crural defect is noticed, the front throat is activated, and a foremost crural fix is performed for little defects or back dissection and fix for bigger defects with rise of the throat to acquire good presentation. If complete dissection of the columns is played out, the fix will be pressure-free. Forceful hiatal crural investigation and fix have been shown to conceivably diminish the rate of band reoperations for immovable reflux, prolapse, and pocket augmentation.

Presentation and position of the band

The choice of the band size relies upon the thickness of the upper stomach and perigastric fat. The vast majority of the patients can have the littler size of each band brand accessible in the United States. As far as we can tell, the patients that typically require a bigger band size are men with a higher body mass list with thicker tissues.

Contingent upon the band type, arrangement on the back table needs to be performed. The Lap-Band AP (Allergan, Irvine, California) requires preparing with saline to suction the air from the framework. The Realize band (Ethicon Endosurgery, Cincinnati, Ohio) just requires yearning of the air until the inflatable is purged completely.

The band is embedded into the midsection through the 15mm trocar. After the band is inside the midsection, the band is gotten through the back esophagogastric burrow. The Lap-Band (Allergan) is pulled from the finish of the tubing rather than the Realize band (Ethicon Endosurgery), which is pulled from the stitch circle appended to the band side. Sometimes the retroperitoneal tissue catches on the band, but for the most part, slides generally simple.

So as to bolt the Lap-Band, the tubing tag is taken care of through the locking system of the band, and the band is bolted. The Realize band conclusion is achieved by embeddings the dissector through the band's clasp opening to get a handle on the end fold, which is gotten through the clasp. The bolted band ought not to be tight on the stomach but instead ought to have the option to turn freely around the upper stomach. If the band seems cozy or doesn't pivot easily, the band needs to be unfastened and more perigastric fat must be extracted.

Anteriorly, a plication of the fundus underneath the band to the upper gastric pocket is needed. Gastrogastric stitching over the band is completed with a perpetual stitch material (Figure 5). The plication ought to be without pressure to prevent any hazard for band disintegration. The plication starts at the more prominent curvature, as far to one side as could be expected under the circumstances. A bended needle is preferred to guarantee secure "nibbles" of tissue between the seromuscular layer of the fundus and the pocket. These lines defensively tunnelate the foremost band, aside from at the area of the clasp, to limit the danger of pressure and conceivable disintegration. The band should lie without strain within the passage to take into account filling during the adjustments. Normally the plication can be cultivated with a few intruded on stitches.

If there is excess floppy fundus beneath the band, an extra plication stitch can be put to fix the more noteworthy curvature fundus to the more steady lesser curvature underneath the band. This stitch needs to be set away and underneath from the band to maintain a strategic distance from tightening and pressure on the band front gastric burrowing. The free finish of the band tubing is gotten out through the 15mm port in anticipation of an obsession with the port framework.

Primary concern

After a time of development of method, the standards flaccida approach has been built up with the formation of a little upper gastric pocket, principally anteriorly, and the dissection on the lesser curvature of the stomach, including the neurovascular heap of the lesser omentum. Stitch obsession of the foremost mass of the stomach, with gastrogastric stitches, is performed to balance out the band anteriorly.

CHAPTER TWENTY-THREE: GASTRIC BAND HYPNOSIS (TIGHTENING)

The band embedded around the stomach is a slight, empty silicone elastic ring, which is joined by a little, meager cylinder. The band is embedded emptied to fit around the stomach, and it is later loaded up with a saline answer to modify the snugness of the band around the organ. This whole procedure is rehashed a few times during the treatment, and it is known as a gastric band adjustment. The gastric banding methodology is the main flexible weight-misfortune surgery accessible in the United States, making it adjustable for every person.

Around four to about a month and a half after the surgery, patients may experience their first band adjustment. The American Society for Metabolic and Bariatric Surgery characterize adjustments as "the implantation of saline for gadget fixing or withdrawal of saline for gadget relaxing by means of an entrance port to change or modify the size of the customizable gastric prohibitive gadget. The need for adjustments depend on clinical appraisal of the patient's craving, satiety, dietary intake, portion size, weight misfortune/gain, and related signs or indications of expected intricacies."

How Are Gastric Band Adjustments Performed?

The adjustments are made without the need for surgery and are led in a procedure that takes around 10 minutes. The cylinder embedded nearby the elastic band likewise incorporates a little port situated just underneath the skin that is utilized to fill the ring with saline and increment the measure of food and caloric limitation. The port is imperceptible and must be felt when pushed by the doctor. During the adjustment procedure, the doctor will utilize a needle to infuse or pull back saline arrangements from the band.

To swell the band and make it closer, the clinical expert will embed more arrangements, while if the band needs to be freer, the expert will expel some saline to reduce the limitation. This framework permits the surgery to be customizable to the patient's individual needs, just as to be reversible if needed. While right after the surgery there are standard adjustment plans, as the patient loses weight, the gastric band adjustments can be made varying, as per the doctor's proposals.

Who Performs Gastric Band Adjustments?

As indicated by The American Society for Metabolic and Bariatric Surgery, so as to satisfy the Global

Credentialing Requirements and be approved to lead gastric band adjustments, a doctor needs to have educational preparing through a gastric band instructional class that, at any rate, incorporates patient determination standards, careful arrangement, surgery, early postoperative management, evaluation of postoperative patient/band adjustment contemplations, adjustment conventions, release directions, long haul dietary and conduct support, long haul inconvenience acknowledgment, appraisal, and management just as training of access port adjustment.

Likewise, doctors additionally need to take an interest in clinical preparation in a preceptor program if accessible or, as a substitute, in a preceptor program followed by directed clinical preparation with an experienced provider. The society includes that for doctor extenders as of now performing gastric band adjustments, the rules that fulfill the credentialing prerequisites remember having just performed adjustments for a bariatric surgery practice for at least a half year, having documentation of 50 adjustments performed, and documentation by an experienced provider of the doctor extender's capacity to perform adjustments.

CHAPTER TWENTY-FOUR: GASTRIC BAND HYPNOSIS (REMOVAL)

A gastric band is fitted when a patient is classed as significant and has a body mass file of more than 40 or more than 35 with weight-related health confusions. Gastric band tasks are proposed to be reversible with the stomach coming back to its original size once the band is expelled. There can be various reasons why patients later decide to have the band expelled, including arriving at their ideal weight, health difficulties, or pregnancy.

Why expel the band?

Before patients at first have their gastric band fitted, they are encouraged to save it forever. This is to keep up their weight misfortune and furthermore because the expulsion activity conveys expanded dangers than the original strategy. Anyway, sometimes there are situations when it is in the patients eventual benefits to expel the band. Sometimes inconveniences with the original surgery will make patients need the band removing. The band is made of a soft plastic, anyway it is as yet an outside body and for certain patients, this can prompt the band to get contaminated. In different patients, the band will consistently rub against the stomach, which will dissolve it after some time. If anti-toxins don't work, then in both of these situations, the band should be expelled.

A few people choose to have their band evacuated for personal reasons. Some accepted their weight issues were because of emotional issues and to keep up a healthy weight would need to manage these issues first.

Pregnancy is additionally a time when ladies may need the band removing. This can be because of both morning ailment and getting enough supplements to the infant while it is in the belly. Patients are encouraged not to have the band supplanted until after they have completed bosom taking care of, to make sure that both mother and infant are getting all the supplements they require.

Evacuation of the band

A gastric band can be evacuated whenever after the activity, although removing the band can make the patient beginning recovering weight. At the point when a gastric band is expelled, the patient's stomach will return to the size it was before the activity. If the patient at that point returns to their old eating habits, they will begin putting weight on.

If the band was fitted utilizing laparoscopic (keyhole) surgery it is conceivable to expel it similarly. Be that as it may, if this bombs open surgery should be performed to evacuate the band. Open surgery requires any longer recuperation time for the patient.

Main concern

Studies have discovered that after gastric band expulsion, 88% of people put on weight. Numerous people found that they needed the gastric band to initially lose weight and to keep up their healthy weight. As gastric band evacuation surgery conveys expanded dangers than the original surgery, it's anything but a choice to be trifled with.

CHAPTER TWENTY-FIVE: GUIDED MEDITATIONS FOR MINDFUL EATING

As we as a whole realize, sustenance is one of the principal establishments of our physical and mental prosperity. Notwithstanding, something has marginally changed in the most recent decade as we are living out a relationship with food in the incorrect way.

Because of internet-based life, because of the thin models we see online constantly, we regularly trash food as it is our main adversary. The outcome? We live our sustenance more as a hindrance than an opportunity to sustain ourselves and deal with ourselves. Reasonably it is realized that it isn't right, but it is significantly more difficult to make a genuine change. Have you at any point known about Mindful Eating to achieve this goal in the field of sustenance?

What is mindful eating?

Mindful eating implies eating consciously and comprises of knowing impeccably the qualities of what we are going to eat while getting a charge out of the experience of food with every one of our senses and therefore have an increasingly legitimate and healthy relationship with food.

Consider the last time you ate something like a treat and your thought about how that treatment was made, what are its fundamental highlights and focus on its shading, smell, and taste. We wager this never happened, right?

Sometimes we use food as solace as a way to mend our emotional injuries; different times we eat because we need to, similar to it was our obligation for the afternoon. This is so off-base and makes a misshaped thought of what food truly is. In addition, if we need to lose some weight, we frequently accuse foods to our most recent increases while our habits ought to be the one to manage and change.

Mindful eating can help us understand which food we truly prefer, what we need in some specific moments of the day, and to recognize genuine nourishment from the moments when that food speaks to different emotions (for example, the need for affection). Mindful eating is fundamentally a powerful different sort of meditation, a training that is done gradually, and this encourages a ton to get mindful of the genuine moments of craving and satiety.

Instructions to rehearse mindful eating

A down to earth exercise to begin with mindful eating is

comprised of a wide range of steps that mean to actuate and stir our senses and our mindfulness. To start with, when we sit before our meal, how about we focus on our body reactions to it and take a couple of full breaths to actuate a condition of attention and focus on what we are doing in that specific moment. For this initial segment is so important to kill your cell phone and every one of your notifications, turn the TV off and indeed be available at this very moment as you would do in a meditation meeting.

From that point forward, you can welcome your attention to what you see: how does the food we are eating resemble? What are its shape and hues? How about we attempt to depict what we have before us. The time has come to enact the sense of smell, we see the aroma by bringing the food close to the nose and attempt to comprehend what we like preferred or less over that smell. If we eat a natural product or something to take with our hands, we can likewise utilize contact, it will give us numerous physical sensations. A good thought is to have a go at envisioning the food we are going to eat in its normal setting. How, for instance, a natural product grew up gratitude to water, sun, cherishing caring motions and how it wound up in your dish right there before you prepared to acquire its energies and properties your body. This is an incredible way to turn out to be increasingly mindful of our planet also, progressively grateful and progressively open to recognize how nature is dealing with us from numerous points of view.

At last, we actuate our taste. As we bite, we attempt to see how the taste changes inside our mouth, we should focus on the way of food and on how it will arrive at our organs and feed us from within in a characteristic compelling way. At long last, we can inquire as to whether we feel completely fulfilled from our meal if our body has gotten the right measure of food or what drives us to keep eating. Obviously we should utilize some fundamental guidelines like eating more frequently, however less during the day, picking characteristic foods and evade voraciously consuming food, one of the riskiest habits of our cutting edge life.

Advantages of mindful eating

If you are captivated yet you don't have the foggiest idea why you should depend on mindful eating, here comes a rundown of the primary advantages of this training:

- You become progressively mindful of what you eat
- You will figure out how your body reacts to specific foods and situations
- You will recognize the importance of nature in our lives
- You will turn out to be progressively grateful for what you have
- You will forget about some stress from the day by day schedule
- You will make a healthy habit
- You will improve your processing

- You will discover that food isn't the foe. Bad habits are!

If mindful eating despite everything sounds somewhat unreasonably precarious for you, simplify the exercise we enrolled previously and make your own! You could do it when you have a bite or breakfast, beginning with something somewhat simpler and convenient. You will realize that it will be a genuine tangible encounter, you will see impressions that you may never have felt identified with food and your body and will change your relationship with food and sustenance for good!

CONCLUSION

Are You Sick and Tired of Struggling to Lose Weight? What's more, Wish there was a Simple Way to Shed Pounds Effortlessly Without Dangerous Gastric Bypass Surgery?

What's more, You Can Do it WITHOUT Crash Dieting, Feeling Deprived, or Risking Your Health with Invasive Surgery!

Dear Friend,

It's no mishap that you're perusing this book right at this point. You're longing for at last shedding the extra pounds that have been tormenting you for a considerable length of time... perhaps decades!

You're not the only one! Many people simply like you the world over consider what it resembles to dispose of their undesirable weight, glance incredible in a bathing suit or sundress... what's more, feel healthy, energetic, and progressively alive!

In the U.S. alone, over 60% of grown-ups are viewed as overweight. These are dedicated, dynamic people simply like you... what's more, regardless of what they do, they just can't shed the extra weight and keep it off!

The principal thing you need to comprehend is that your weight issues aren't your shortcoming! The human body is hard-wired to gather and store extra fat, especially as we age. This filled in as a characteristic endurance component a huge number of years back. Be that as it may, today, it can bargain your self-regard, your satisfaction, and even your health!

Yet, our hereditary qualities haven't exactly found our cutting edge lifestyles. Thus people like you and me regularly go through years fighting with our bodies' programming, and it tends to be nothing shy of disappointing!

Inform me as to whether any of these ring a bell:

You've spent incalculable hours in the rec center every week beating away on high-impact exercise machines... be that as it may, regardless of how strongly you exercise, you can't drop a solitary pound.

You've had a go at constraining your portions at mealtimes, yet you simply wind up compensating for it (to say the very least) with tidbits when your meals simply don't fulfill you.

You've become tied up with each trend diet out there, regardless of how strange it sounds, basically because you're edgy to lose weight and appreciate a trim, hot figure.

You've abandoned your weight misfortune goals at any

rate once out of sheer disappointment until you look in the mirror one day and scarcely perceive the person gazing back at you!

You've needed to manage people disclosing to you things like, "You simply need to eat less" and "Simply exercise more, and you'll be fine"... even though these people have never battled with weight every day in their lives.

You've endured a long time of "low fat" foods and appalling eating routine meals... until you finally surrender in disappointment because you can't take not eating genuine food!

Abstains from food simply don't work for a great many people. They rely upon sheer willpower, also, regardless of how decided you are, keeping up a restrictive, unfulfilling diet won't keep going forever.

What's more, although exercise is a basic component of ideal health, it won't get you looking flying so far in the new year. You can unfortunately spend a limited number of hours seven days on torment gadgets, for example, ellipticals, treadmills, and step steppers. You have a life, and exercise essentially can't occupy the entirety of your time!

It's a little marvel, at that point, that...

A large number of people like you turn to Gastric Band Hypnosis to solve their weight loss problem!

Positive Affirmations for Weight Loss

Stop emotional eating and develop healthy eating habits. Learn how to lose weight easily and improve your mental health with hypnosis and guided meditation

By:Martin Eland

INTRODUCTION

The entranced individual seems to notice just the correspondences of the trance specialist and ordinarily reacts in an uncritical, programmed style while overlooking all parts of the environment other than those brought up by the subliminal specialist. In a sleep-inducing state, an individual will, in general, observe, feel, smell, and in any case, see as per the trance specialist's suggestions, even though these suggestions might be in apparent inconsistency to the real upgrades present in the environment. The impacts of hypnosis are not constrained to tangible change; even the subject's memory and consciousness of self might be adjusted by suggestion. The impacts of the suggestions might be broadened (post hypnotically) into the subject's resulting waking action.

Regardless of whether you're hoping to improve your general wellbeing or basically thin down for summer, burning off abundance fat can be very testing.

Notwithstanding diet and exercise, different components can impact weight and fat loss.

Fortunately, there are many basic advances you can take

to increase fat burning, rapidly and without any problem.

Here are some of the most ideal ways to consume fat rapidly and advance weight loss.

These tips are general ones to support you. Progressively significant hints will be talked about in chapters later in this book.

1. Start Strength Training

Strength training is a sort of exercise that expects you to get your muscles against the opposition. It assembles muscle mass and increases strength.

Most generally, strength training includes lifting weights to gain muscle after some time.

Examination has discovered strength training to have various medical advantages, particularly with regards to burning fat.

In one study, strength training reduced instinctive fat in 78 people with a metabolic condition. Instinctive fat is a sort of hazardous fat that encompasses the organs in the belly.

Another study showed that 12 weeks of strength training combined with aerobic exercise was increasingly successful at lessening body fat and belly fat than aerobic exercise alone.

Opposition training may likewise help preserve without fat mass, which can increase the number of calories your body consumes very still.

As indicated by one survey, ten weeks of obstruction training could help increase calories consumed very still by 7% and may reduce fat weight by 4 pounds (1.8 kg).

Doing body-weight exercises, lifting weights, or utilizing rec center gear are a couple of simple ways to begin with strength training.

Strength training has been appeared to increase resting vitality use and reduce belly fat, particularly when joined with aerobic exercise.

2. Follow a High-Protein Diet

Counting more protein-rich foods in your diet is a compelling way to reduce your craving and consume progressively fat.

Different investigations have discovered that eating all the more top-notch protein is related to a lower danger of belly fat.

One study additionally showed that a high-protein diet could assist preserve with muscling mass and digestion during weight loss.

Increasing your protein intake may likewise increase sentiments of totality, decline craving, and reduce calorie intake to help in weight loss.

Have a go at fusing a couple of servings of high-protein foods into your diet every day to help amp up fat burning.

A few instances of protein-rich foods incorporate meat, seafood, eggs, vegetables, and dairy items.

Eating more protein might be related to a lower danger of belly fat. Expanding your protein intake can diminish craving, lower calorie intake, and preserve muscle mass.

3. Press in More Sleep

Hitting the sack somewhat prior or setting your morning timer somewhat later can assist boost with fat burning and prevent weight gain.

A few investigations have discovered a relationship between getting enough rest and weight loss.

One study of 68,183 ladies showed that the individuals who dozed five or fewer hours out of each night over a time of 16 years were bound to gain weight than the individuals who dozed for longer than seven hours out of every night.

Another study showed that better rest quality and getting in any event seven hours of rest for every night increased the probability of fruitful weight loss by 33% in 245 ladies who took a crack at a six-month weight loss program.

Other examination shows that an absence of rest may add to modifications in hunger hormones, increased craving, and a greater danger of stoutness.

Even though everybody needs a different measure of rest, most investigations have discovered that getting, in any event, seven hours of rest for each night is related to the most advantages with regards to body weight.

Adhere to a standard rest plan, limit your intake of caffeine, and limit your utilization of electronic gadgets before bed to help bolster a sound rest cycle.

Getting enough rest might be related to diminished craving and appetite, just as a lower danger of weight gain.

4. Add Vinegar to Your Diet

Vinegar is notable for its wellbeing advancing properties.

Notwithstanding its likely impacts on heart wellbeing and blood sugar control, expanding your intake of vinegar may help knock up fat burning, as indicated by some exploration.

One study found that expending 1–2 tablespoons (15–30 ml) of vinegar every day reduced people's body weight, belly fat, and normal waist circumference over a

12-week time frame.

Devouring vinegar has likewise been appeared to upgrade sentiments of completion and reduce hunger.

Another small study of 11 people showed that adding vinegar to the diet reduced daily calorie intake by up to 275 calories.

It's anything but difficult to join vinegar into your diet. For instance, numerous people weaken apple juice vinegar with water and drink it as a refreshment a couple of times for each day with dinners.

Notwithstanding, if drinking vinegar straight doesn't sound engaging, you can likewise utilize it to make dressings, sauces, and marinades.

Vinegar may help increase sentiments of completion, decline calorie intake, and lower body fat.

5. Eat More Healthy Fats

Even though it might appear to be irrational, expanding your intake of solid fats may help prevent weight gain and assist you with keeping up sentiments of totality.

Fat requires a significant period to process and can help moderate the purging of the stomach, which can reduce craving and appetite.

One study found that following a Mediterranean diet

wealthy in sound fats from olive oil and nuts was related to a lower danger of weight gain contrasted with a low-fat diet.

Another small study found that when people on a weight loss diet took two tablespoons (30 ml) of coconut oil every day, they lost more belly fat than the individuals who were given soybean oil.

Then, unfortunate kinds of fat like trans fats have appeared to increase body fat, waist circumference, and belly fat in humans and creatures.

Olive oil, coconut oil, avocados, nuts, and seeds are only a couple of instances of solid sorts of fat that may effectively affect fat burning.

Notwithstanding, remember that solid fat is still high in calories, so moderate the amount you devour. Rather than eating increasingly fat by and large, have a go at trading the unfortunate fats in your diet for these substantial fat assortments.

Fat is processed gradually, so eating it can help reduce hunger. A higher intake of solid fats is related to a lower danger of weight gain and diminished belly fat.

6. Drink Healthier Beverages

Trading out sugar-improved beverages for some more advantageous choices is probably the most straightforward way to increase fat burning.

For instance, sugar-improved refreshments like pop and squeeze are stuffed with calories and offer minimal health benefits.

Liquor is likewise high in calories and has the additional impact of lowering your restraints, making you bound to indulge.

Studies have discovered that devouring both sugar-improved drinks and liquor is related to a more serious danger of belly fat.

Constraining your intake of these refreshments can help reduce your calorie intake and hold your waistline under wraps.

Instead, pick without calorie refreshments like water or green tea.

In one small, 12-week study, drinking 17 ounces (500 ml) of water before dinners increased weight loss by 4.4 pounds (2 kg), contrasted with a benchmark group.

Green tea is another incredible alternative. It contains caffeine and is wealthy in cell reinforcements, the two of which may assist increase with fatting burning and upgrade digestion.

For example, one study in 12 grown-ups showed that green tea extricate increased fat burning by 12% contrasted with a fake treatment.

Exchanging even only a couple of servings of fatty

drinks for a glass of water or some green tea is a straightforward way to advance fat burning.

Sugar-improved refreshments and mixed beverages might be related with a higher danger of belly fat. Green tea and water have been appeared to increase weight loss and fat burning.

7. Top off on Fiber

Solvent fiber ingests water and travels through the stomach related tract gradually, helping you feel more full for more.

As per a few investigations, expanding your intake of high-fiber foods may ensure against weight gain and fat aggregation.

One study of 1,114 grown-ups found that for every 10-gram increase in dissolvable fiber intake every day, members lost 3.7% of their belly fat over a five-year time frame, even with no different changes in diet or exercise.

Another survey likewise found that expanding fiber intake advanced sentiments of completion and diminished appetite. Indeed, an increase of 14 grams of fiber for each day was related to a 10% reduction in calorie intake.

That, yet it was additionally connected to about 4.4 pounds (2 kg) of weight loss over a four-month time span.

Organic products, vegetables, vegetables, entire grains, nuts, and seeds are a couple of instances of high-fiber foods that can boost fat burning and weight loss.

A higher intake of fiber might be related to fat loss, diminished calorie intake, and greater weight loss.

8. Cut Down on Refined Carbs

Diminishing your intake of refined sugars may assist you with losing additional fat.

During preparing, refined grains are deprived of their wheat and germ, bringing about the last item that is low in fiber and supplements.

Refined carbs additionally will have a higher glycemic file, which can cause spikes and crashes in blood sugar levels, bringing about increased appetite.

Studies show that a diet high in refined carbs might be related to increased belly fat.

Alternately, a diet high in entire grains has been related to a lower body mass record and body weight, in addition to a smaller waist circumference.

One study in 2,834 people likewise showed that those with higher intakes of refined grains would, in general, have a higher measure of ailment advancing belly fat. In contrast, the individuals who ate all the more entire grains would, in general, have a lower sum.

For the best outcomes, reduce your intake of refined carbs from cakes, handled foods, pasta, white slices of bread, and breakfast grains. Supplant them with entire grains, for example, whole wheat, quinoa, buckwheat, grain, and oats.

Refined carbs are low in fiber and supplements. They may increase craving and cause spikes and crashes in blood sugar levels. Devouring refined carbs has additionally been related to increased belly fat.

9. Increase Your Cardio

Cardio, otherwise called aerobic exercise, is one of the most widely recognized types of exercise and is characterized as an exercise that specifically prepares the heart and lungs.

Adding cardio to your routine might be one of the best ways to improve fat burning.

For instance, one audit of 16 examinations found that the more aerobic exercise people got, the more belly fat they lost.

Different investigations have discovered that aerobic exercise can increase muscle mass and reduction in belly fat, waist circumference, and body fat.

Most examination suggests between 150–300 minutes of moderate to overwhelming exercise weekly, or about 20–40 minutes of cardio every day.

Running, strolling, cycling, and swimming are only a couple of instances of some cardio exercises that can assist ignite with fatting and launch weight loss.

Studies show that the more aerobic exercise people get, the more belly fat they will, in general, lose. Cardio may likewise help reduce waist circumference, lower body fat, and increase muscle mass.

10. Drink Coffee

Caffeine is an essential fixing in pretty much every fat-burning enhancement, and in light of current circumstances.

The caffeine found in coffee goes about as a focal sensory system energizer, increases digestion, and boosts the breakdown of fatty acids.

Indeed, examinations show that caffeine intake can briefly increase vitality use and improve digestion by 3–11%.

One huge study with more than 58,000 people found that increased caffeine intake was related to less weight gain over 12 years.

Another study found that higher caffeine intake was connected to a higher pace of progress with weight loss upkeep among 2,623 people.

To augment the medical advantages of coffee, avoid the

cream and sugar. Instead, appreciate it dark or with a small measure of milk to prevent the additional calories from piling up.

Coffee contains caffeine, which can increase the breakdown of fat and raise digestion. Studies show that higher caffeine intake might be related with greater weight loss.

11. Attempt High-Intensity Interval Training (HIIT)

High-intensity interval training, otherwise called HIIT, is a type of exercise that sets snappy explosions of movement with short recuperation periods to keep your pulse raised.

Studies show that HIIT can be extraordinarily compelling at inclining up fat burning and advancing weight loss.

One study found that youngsters performing HIIT for 20 minutes three times weekly lost a normal of 4.4 pounds (2 kg) of body fat over a 12-week duration, even with no different changes to their diet or lifestyle.

They additionally encountered a 17% decrease in belly fat, just as a significant diminishing in waist circumference.

HIIT may likewise assist you with burning more calories in a shorter measure of time than different types of cardio.

As indicated by one study, performing HIIT helped people wreck to 30% more calories than different sorts of exercise, for example, cycling or running, in a similar measure of time.

A simple way to begin with HIIT is to shift back and forth between strolling and running or running for 30 seconds, one after another.

You can likewise cycle between exercises like burpees, push-ups, or squats with a brief rest period in the middle.

HIIT can assist increase with fatting burning and consume more calories in a shorter measure of time than different types of exercise.

12. Add Probiotics to Your Diet

Probiotics are a kind of useful microorganisms found in your stomach related tract that have appeared to improve numerous parts of well-being.

The microorganisms in your gut have been appeared to assume a job in everything from insusceptibility to emotional wellness.

Expanding your intake of probiotics through either food or enhancements may likewise help fire up fat burning and monitor your weight.

One audit of 15 investigations showed that people who took probiotics experienced significantly bigger decreases in body weight, fat rate, and body mass record contrasted with the individuals who received a fake treatment.

Another small study showed that taking probiotic supplements helped people following a high-fat, unhealthy diet prevent fat and weight gain (.

Certain strains of probiotics in the family Lactobacillus might be particularly viable at helping weight and fat loss.

One study showed that eating yogurt containing either Lactobacillus fermentum or Lactobacillus amylovorus microbes reduced body fat by 3–4% (52).

Taking enhancements is a speedy and simple way to get in a concentrated portion of probiotics consistently.

On the other hand, you can take a stab at adding some probiotic-rich foods to your diet, for example, kefir, tempeh, natto, a fermented tea, kimchi, and sauerkraut.

Taking probiotic supplements or expanding your intake of probiotics through food sources may help reduce body weight and fat rate.

13. Increase Your Iron Intake

Iron is a significant mineral that has numerous

fundamental functions in the body.

Similarly, as with different supplements, for example, iodine, an insufficiency in iron may affect the strength of your thyroid organ. This small organ in your neck secretes hormones that direct your digestion.

Numerous examinations have discovered that low levels of iron in the body might be related to impaired thyroid function and an interruption in the creation of thyroid hormones.

Basic indications of hypothyroidism, or diminished thyroid function, incorporate shortcoming, fatigue, the brevity of breath, and weight gain.

Mainly, an insufficiency in iron can cause side effects like fatigue, unsteadiness, cerebral pains, and brevity of breath.

Rewarding iron inadequacy can permit your digestion to work all the more effectively and ward off fatigue to increase your activity level.

One study even found that when 21 ladies were treated for iron insufficiency, they encountered decreases in body weight, waist circumference, and body mass list.

Lamentably, numerous people don't get enough iron in their diets.

Ladies, babies, kids, veggie lovers, and vegans are all at a higher danger of iron inadequacy.

Make sure to join a lot of iron-rich foods in your diet to help meet your iron needs and keep up your digestion and vitality levels.

You can discover iron in meat, poultry, seafood, fortified grains and oats, verdant green vegetables, dried foods grown from the ground.

A lack of iron might be related to impaired thyroid function and can cause indications like fatigue and brevity of breath. One study found that rewarding iron lack supported in weight loss.

14. Give Intermittent Fasting a Shot

Irregular fasting is a diet design that includes cycling between times of eating and fasting.

Examination shows that irregular fasting may help to upgrade both weight loss and fat loss.

One audit took a gander at the impacts of discontinuous fasting, including exchange day fasting — a strategy that includes switching back and forth between days of fasting and eating typically.

They found that other day fasting over a time of 3–12 weeks reduced body weight by up to 7% and diminished body fat by as much as 12 pounds (5.5 kg).

Another small study showed that eating just during an eight-hour window every day helped decline fat mass and keep up muscle mass when joined with opposition training.

There are a few different sorts of discontinuous fasting, including someplace you eat just on specific days of the week and others where eating is confined to specific hours of the day.

Well-known kinds of irregular fasting incorporate Eat Stop Eat, the Warrior Diet, the 16/8 technique, and the 5:2 diet.

Discover a variety that fits in with your timetable and lifestyle, and don't be reluctant to analyze to discover what works best for you.

Discontinuous fasting has been appeared to reduce body weight and body fat and may assist preserve with muscling mass when joined with opposition training.

CHAPTER ONE: WEIGHT LOSS IDEAS TO GET YOU INSPIRED

You settled on it here-the choice to lose weight! This implies mindfulness is kicking in! This is significant for motivation, weight loss, and well-being. Being solid and dynamic is essential!

Our bodies were intended to move, not be stationary. For weight loss, the achievement of your journey depends on your capacity to remain inspired all through.

Motivation is simple from the start. Clutching it might raise a little test. It will be ideal if you realize this is typical. You will have days where motivation is at its unequaled high, and different days where motivation is at an unprecedented low.

We'll investigate the absolute best thoughts on motivation to lose weight and why we lose motivation effectively along the weight loss journey.

Motivation and Inspiration for losing weight

There are fluctuated explanations behind needing to lose weight. The one basic factor: Everyone needs motivation.

One recommendation:

Motivation comes a little simpler when you decide the purpose behind needing to lose weight.

What is/are your rousing components for losing weight? It is essential to comprehend your "why," regardless of how small.

Losing weight, even only 5% of your weight, can help:

- Improve blood sugar
- Reduce the danger of coronary illness
- Lower cholesterol
- Reduce joint agony
- Reduce the danger of specific tumors

As somebody who has experienced this journey, I can reveal that it will require consistent revives of motivation.

Motivation is extremely solid first and foremost; motivation begins to shift when the outcomes aren't quick. The outcomes require some serious energy, and your motivation is vital to get you there.

Motivation is the thing that kicks you off. Propensity is the thing that props you up.

Normal weight loss motivation battles

The absence of motivation is normal for some reasons. Motivation can trigger various feelings, making it difficult to get spurred. A portion of the regular motivation battles that people face:

Unsupportive social environment

Your social environment is your physical and social setting (home, family, companions, and so on.).

Many don't understand the significance and impact of a social environment. If you are attempting to jump destined for success and hear something like "gracious, you don't have to do that, how about we go out and get frozen yogurt," your motivation to make the best choice is will probably be affected.

Bunches of difficult work for moderate outcomes

At the point when you work out five times every week and cautiously check your calories, you usually need to see multiple pounds gone. If it's not too much trouble, remember that ordinary and solid weight loss midpoints 2 pounds for every week; around 3500 calories consumed implies one pound lost.

Wounds

Many experience the ill effects of wounds that reduce their capacity to exercise; notwithstanding, thought for low effect exercise and exercise modifications ought to be given.

Furthermore, examining affirmed exercises with your primary care physician is useful. Exercise can occur with a physical issue; don't lose motivation!

Longings

You will pine for, and it is alright! Indeed, even the most beneficial people have longings. At the point when longings strike, be mindful of the hankering and the bit.

Longing for treats? Prepare them at home with the goal that you can modify and control the formula for your objective!

Solid food is costly

There is a touch of truth and somewhat of a lie here. Healthy food can be somewhat costly; in any case, if you eat all the more a plant-based diet (organic products, vegetables, grains, and so forth.), the expenses won't soar.

Absence of time for working out

If losing weight is truly what you are decided to achieve, at that point, time must be found. You need to calendar and organize your day to day to incorporate an exercise.

For a considerable length of time that you can't, settle on decisions that power somewhat more development:

Park at the back of the parking area and go for a more drawn out stroll into the store, use the stairwell rather than the lift, do squats while cooking, and additionally sit-ups during business breaks.

The significance of mindfulness for motivation and weight loss

Be straightforward with yourself, how frequently have you eaten something without really pondering what you were taking care of yourself?

Mindfulness assumes a significant job in our everyday choices, particularly the decisions in regards to our wellbeing. Here are mindfulness contemplations that will help propel you to lose weight.

Before, we were instructed what to eat and what not to eat; in any case, there was no direction on the most proficient method to choose and devour, which eventually adds to weight issues.

As a rule, people have a solid misguided judgment about food and its motivation in our lives and wellbeing. This makes undesirable propensities that add to weight gain.

The significance of mindfulness in this journey is urgent to your weight loss achievement.

Investigate this article to become familiar with mindful eating:

17 Ways to inspire yourself to lose weight

1. Love and appreciation

Love moves motivation, and motivation takes care of appreciation.

Cherishing yourself inspires you to value our body and all the things that it can do. Thankfulness for the body improves body picture, and gratefulness for body picture prompts weight loss motivation.

2. Mindfulness

As talked about above, mindfulness is vital for progress. Being mindful guarantees that you know about your "why," the purpose behind beginning your weight loss journey, and are committed to using sound judgment that helps your definitive objective.

Mindfulness likewise keeps you mindful of food decisions, social settings, and procedures/progress.

3. Be submitted

The motivation for weight loss will endure if you are not dedicated. Doing an open duty will help consider you responsible and improve motivation.

4. Get a coach/Accountability partner

Having a guide as well as an accountability partner will help with motivation. Having somebody that rouses you and has confidence in you will boost motivation.

5. Creatures help persuade

Getting a pooch will increase development. Pooches need to head outside and play. A pooch can be an accountability partner!

Not exclusively will they make you move, they are wonderful to help creatures.

6. Objective setting

You know your "why," and now you're prepared to begin. What are your objectives? It is safe to say that they are practical?

As talked about over a normal of 2 pounds a week is ordinary and sound weight loss. Defining objectives like "I plan on losing 15 pounds in a week" will bring about an absence of motivation toward the week's end.

7. Take on a steady speed

The weight loss journey is a lifestyle change journey. This doesn't occur within a couple of days. Propensities enjoy time to delay. Try not to lose trust!

8. Flawlessness doesn't exist, and setbacks will occur

Try not to be so difficult on yourself. Be patient and love yourself through this procedure. This isn't a simple journey. Expect a couple of setbacks as you change and get into the section.

9. Try not to focus on the end, set them on every day

What I mean is center around the journey, not the ultimate objective.

If you are attempting to lose 50 pounds, concentrating on that number will inspire you at first; nonetheless, it will cause the absence of motivation later due to being overpowered about the period.

Rather, center around your day by day objectives.

10. Fuse an arrangement that accommodates your day-to-day life

Everybody has different obligations and different

explanations behind losing weight. One arrangement doesn't work from everybody.

Construct your own arrangement, one that you can fit into your consistent life.

Mindfulness is key here and helps keep you spurred. Being mindful of your day to day and fusing a weight loss plan is significant.

A couple of suggestions:

• Reduce the number of calories you eat. Keep a food diary and track everything.

• Make smaller plates with smaller segments. Part control is significant.

• Reduce your undesirable bite and sugar intake. Sugar can raise fiasco.

• Stay away from southern style/seared foods.

• Eat plenty of products of the soil.

11. Try not to gauge yourself every day

This is a tremendous NO. Saying something once every week and monitoring progress is the thing that you need. Gauging yourself once a day is perhaps the quickest way to lose motivation.

Keep in mind, solid weight loss midpoints 2 pounds for

each week.

12. Try not to concentrate 100% on the scale

The scale is only one way to follow the movement, and even in that, exceptional thought must be given.

You may have jumped on the scale two weeks back and have shed 15 pounds. This week you may see 5 pounds gained.

If you transformed fat into muscle, this will occur, don't lose motivation! This is something to be thankful for! It implies you are burning fat and building muscle. Building muscle implies conditioning up.

13. Celebrate and prize yourself!

At the point when you arrive at an objective, celebrate! Offer your prosperity with your social environment.

Being upbeat and praising your accomplishment improves motivation.

14. Recruit a coach

It is alright to enlist a professional mentor to help rouse and mentor you toward your weight-loss objective. The mentor doesn't need to be an exercise coach. Think about a dietician or a potential specialist.

15. Use music

Music is a motivation booster without a doubt! Music will assist you with moving and notch, removing the concentration from the demonstration, and permitting gladly to kick in and rouse you!

Exploration directed by the North American Association for the Study of Obesity found that those that tuned in to music while practicing were bound to stay with it than the individuals who didn't.

16. Keep those pants!

You may have some pants that you need to get back into. Keep them! Let them persuade you.

17. Take pictures and record your greatness!

Your body will change as your dietary patterns and exercise propensities change. Snap a photo toward the beginning and consider a photograph each 30 to 60 days. Seeing your improvement will help keep you propelled.

Instructions to get weight loss motivation back when it's lost

You may get yourself 100% persuaded before all else and less roused following a couple of weeks of endeavoring.

Remember that propensities, for the most part, enjoy 21 days to reprieve. If you end up with 0 motivation, in the wake of having been 100% propelled previously, attempt these:

• **Go back to your why**. For what reason did you start? What was the reason?

• **Try resetting your objective**. Possibly your underlying objective was excessively forceful. It's alright to alter and do what works for you.

• **Talk to a mentor/coach**. It is a smart thought to talk about battles with professionals. Many will offer free knowledge and guidance for beginning and remaining on target.

• **Re-consider an accountability partner or potentially gathering**. Being around similarly invested people on your journey can help such a great amount with motivation.

• **Find out if working out is the issue**. Turning out to be separated from everyone else can be somewhat exhausting. Have you considered a gathering wellness class? This returns to being around similarly invested people that are sharing your journey.

• **Get progressively motivational messages**. Words and expressions of certification are so significant. Cherishing yourself and showing restraint toward yourself is at the center of accomplishment for this journey. What about awakening every day to a motivational message that you composed for yourself?

• **Stop contrasting yourself with others**. Weight loss reasons, weight loss motivation, and weight loss journeys are different for everybody. Concentrating on the journey of others removes you from your objectives and achievements. Try not to contrast your advancement and anybody else's.

This is your journey, and you'll do extraordinary!

CHAPTER TWO: HISTORY OF HYPNOTISM

The utilization of hypnosis returns, at any rate, the extent that the Aesculapian 'rest sanctuaries' of Greece of 500bc, which were structured specifically for the treatment of the intellectually sick. Ministers would incite 'rest' utilizing custom and afterward decipher the fantasies of the 'patients,' trying to cast out 'awful' spirits. Taken a gander at unbiasedly, we can see that it is a type of suggestion treatment; however, there are no records to reveal to us how effective or else they were. The cutting edge picture of the trance inducer is affected by an eighteenth-century Austrian physicist by the name of Franz Anton Mesmer (1734 – 1815). Mesmer was liable for practically without any help carrying hypnosis to the consideration of the overall population – just it wasn't called hypnosis at that point, because he named it 'Creature Magnetism.' Mesmer guaranteed that it was the point at which the attractive fields in our bodies got upset or got into a struggle or were streaming the incorrect way that we turned out to be sick. He built up this to some degree peculiar idea after watching a road 'performer' controlling lodestones – magnets – which were at that time totally obscure. Mesmer's crowd were absolutely in wonderment at how his 'performer's wand' would pull in, repulse, and move the lodestones around because they'd never observed something like this. The story has it that this road entertainer informed the group concerning attraction and declared that there is an attraction in all things and everybody, at that point, he started to make suggestions to specific people that if he contacted them with his performer's wand, it would modify the attraction in their bodies so one would tumble to the ground giggling, another would tumble to the ground crying, etc. Incredibly, whatever was recommended really occurred, and it more likely than not been at that point that he concluded that if the course of the attraction wasn't right, at that point, that is the point at which we become sick. Mesmer made plans to explore different avenues regarding the utilization of this astounding marvel in medication, and quickly found that he could deliver evident supernatural occurrence remedies for a wide range of diseases. Mesmer was incredibly fruitful in his remedial undertakings and, in the 1780s, had people lining up at the renowned Paris Salon. He couldn't treat them all and built up some incredibly novel ways to deal with treatment to oblige everyone who looked for his assistance. One of these was to move his attraction to a tree in the patio, basically by contacting it with one of his 'attractive poles'; a significant number of the individuals who talked with him couldn't see him and be coordinated that the following best thing was to touch the polarized tree – they despite everything showed signs of improvement from whatever distressed them.

Another tale strategy he created involved simply a barrel of sand, from which trailed a few ropes; his patients had to lounge around the barrel, clutching one of the ropes to discover alleviation from their indications. Such was the intensity of suggestion before science and instruction had carried their impact to hold up under the western world. It was the renowned American researcher and representative, Benjamin Franklin, who was answerable for blasting Mesmer's air pocket. In 1785, when he was right around 80, he was selected as one of a commission of three by the French Government – Franklin was an extremely well known and regarded figure in France at that point – to explore precisely what Mesmer was evidently ready to do. Indeed, it appears that he saw through it basically promptly and articulated that: "If these people show signs of improvement by any means, at that point they do as such by their own creative mind." obviously, it was a suggestion, as opposed to creative mind yet neither he nor Mesmer himself knew about how amazing the power of suggestion can be, at that time. Even though his strategies fell into unsavoriness after Franklin's denouncement, Mesmer has stayed one of the most critical figures in the field of recuperating; even right up till the present time, people utilize the articulation 'Mesmerized' typically important to be somehow or another transfixed or rendered stable by an outside power. It was really Mesmer who built up hand goes around and close to the body, which numerous people despite everything, accept is one of the insider facts of the hypnotherapist, moving his hands, probably, within the alleged attractive field of his subject. How did Mesmer's Animal Magnetism wind up being called hypnosis? It was a Scottish eye specialist by the name of James Braid (1795-1860) who tried different things with the marvel and authored that name 'Hypnosis' after Hypnos, the Greek great of rest. He named it hypnosis after observing an introduction of Mesmerism in which he constrained a pin underneath the finger-nail of the subject, a little youngster. When she showed not even the smallest indication of inconvenience, he was intrigued to the point that he later completed various analyses for himself and, in the long run, gave the procedure its new, however mistaken name. Afterward, Braid understood his misstep in that it had nothing to do with rest, and he needed to rename it 'mono-idealism' – all out fixation on a single line of reasoning. The open cherished the clearly paranormal nature of the possibility of an artificial rest express that could create energizing wonders. It was, in one way or another, like the stupor express that mediums entered. They would acknowledge no exhausting clinical name as a swap, and hypnosis was here for acceptable. A Frenchman, Emile Coué (1857 – 1926), moved away from customary methodologies and started the utilization of autosuggestion. His most well-known expression was, 'step by step inside and out I am improving and better.' He likewise comprehended the significance of the subject's cooperation in hypnosis. He was an early harbinger of experts who currently guarantee, 'There is nothing of the sort as hypnosis, just self-hypnosis.' The cutting edge acknowledgment of hypnosis in medication that we presently have owes an extraordinary obligation to explore beginning in the 1920s and '30s by pioneer Clark Hull and his then understudy, Milton H. Erickson. Erickson proceeded to turn into the perceived driving expert on clinical hypnosis, and an ace of circuitous hypnosis, who had the option to place an individual into a 'stupor' without referencing the word hypnosis. Erickson's methodology and its subordinates are generally acknowledged as the best procedures. Milton Erickson kicked the bucket in 1980, yet left numerous followers of his work.

The focal marvel of hypnosis is suggestibility, a condition of significantly upgraded openness and responsiveness to suggestions and boosts introduced by the trance specialist. Proper suggestions by the trance inducer can prompt an amazingly wide scope of mental, tangible, and engine reactions from people who are profoundly entranced. By acknowledgment of and reaction to suggestions, the subject can be incited to carry on as though hard of hearing, visually impaired, incapacitated, daydreamed, whimsical, amnesic, or impenetrable to torment or to awkward body stances; also, the subject can show different conduct reactions that the individual in question sees as a sensible or alluring reaction to the circumstance that has been recommended by the subliminal specialist.

One entrancing manifestation that can be evoked from a

subject which has been in a sleep-inducing daze is that of posthypnotic suggestion and conduct; that is, the subject's execution of guidelines and suggestions that were given to him while he was in a stupor. With satisfactory amnesia prompted during the stupor express, the individual won't know about the wellspring of his motivation to play out the educated demonstration. Posthypnotic suggestion, be that as it may, is certifiably not an especially amazing method for controlling conduct compared with an individual's cognizant ability to perform activities.

Numerous subjects appear to be not able to review occasions that happened while they were in profound hypnosis. This "posthypnotic amnesia" can result either immediately from profound hypnosis or a suggestion by the trance inducer while the subject is unconscious. The amnesia may incorporate all the occasions of the stupor state or just chose things, or it might be manifested regarding matters irrelevant to the daze. Proper sleep-inducing suggestions might effectively evacuate posthypnotic amnesia.

Hypnosis has been officially supported as a helpful technique by clinical, mental, dental, and mental relationships all through the world. It has been discovered generally helpful in getting ready people for sedation, improving the medication reaction, and lessening the necessary measurement. In labor, it is especially useful, because it can help mitigate the mother's inconvenience while staying away from sedatives that could disable the youngster's physiological function. Hypnosis has often been utilized in endeavors to quit smoking, and it is exceptionally respected in the administration of, in any case, unmanageable torment, including that of a terminal disease. It is significant in diminishing the basic dread of dental strategies; truth be told, the very people whom dental specialists generally find difficult to treat often react best to sleep-inducing suggestion. In the territory of psychosomatic medication, hypnosis has been utilized in an assortment of ways. Patients have been prepared to unwind and to complete, without the hypnotherapist, exercises that have effectively affected a few types of hypertension, migraines, and functional issue.

Even though the acceptance of hypnosis requires small training and no specific expertise, when utilized with regards to clinical treatment, it may be harming when used by people who do not have the capability and aptitude to treat such issues without the utilization of hypnosis. Then again, hypnosis has been over and again denounced by different clinical affiliations when it is utilized only for motivations behind open diversion, inferable from the peril of unfavorable posthypnotic responses to the methodology. Surely, in such a manner, a few countries have prohibited or constrained business or other open showcases of hypnosis. Also, numerous official courtrooms will not acknowledge declaration from people who have been entranced for reasons for "recuperating" recollections, because such procedures can prompt disarray among minds and recollections.

CHAPTER THREE: WHAT IS HYPNOSIS FOR WEIGHT LOSS?

Many people couldn't want anything more than to accomplish their ideal weight and shape as a way of expanding their certainty and confidence. It is critical to manage any intense subject matters behind their weight issues.

This professionally composed book can help rouse your customers in their mission to accomplish their ideal weight and shape. They will likewise be better outfitted to manage triggers that lead to over or under-eating.

The book tends to issues, for example, fatigue eating, over-enjoying food subtly (for instance, in the evening), family weight, absence of exercise, and imagining themselves experiencing a gastric band strategy to eat less.

There are likewise approaches for customers who need to quick - regardless of whether to lose weight or to detox - and approaches for keeping up that weight loss once it has been accomplished.

A few people might need to eat more advantageous and appreciate increasingly nutritious foods, for example, products of the soil or eat and drink all the more gradually. You can assist your customers with appreciating and enjoy meals that in the past they couldn't endure - just as sail through merriments, for example, Christmas and Thanksgiving that are often connected with immense and visit eating as they appreciate a more advantageous lifestyle and arrive at their objective weight and shape.

The procedure of hypnosis is getting your mind into a state where it can acknowledge a suggestion. During hypnosis, a subject can bring an excursion profound into their subconscious to dispense with convictions and propensities that might be a drawback to his everyday life. This is the reason hypnosis is so mainstream for those trying to lose weight. In any case, it isn't essential to look for and pay for a professional. Most protection designs likewise don't take care of the expense of hypnotherapy too. Attempt to self-entrance yourself to lose additional weight.

Section 1. Entrancing Yourself

1. **Accept**. A significant part of the intensity of hypnosis rests in the way that you have persuaded yourself that you have a way to assume responsibility for your desires. If you don't accept that hypnosis will assist you with changing your sentiments, it will presumably have little impact.

2. **Get settled**. Go to a spot where you are not liable to

be upset. This can be anyplace that hushes up like your bed, a sofa, or an agreeable, comfortable chair. Ensure that your head and neck are bolstered.

Wear loose garments and set up that the temperature is set at an agreeable level.

It's simpler to unwind if you play some delicate music while you self-spellbind, especially something instrumental.

3. **Concentrate on an item**. Discover something in the space to take a gander at and center around, preferably something somewhat above you. Utilize your attention to this article to free your head from all contemplations. Make this item the main thing you are aware of.

4 . **Inhale profoundly as you close your eyes**. Reveal to yourself that your eyelids are getting substantial and permit them to fall tenderly. As you close your eyes, inhale profoundly with a customary musicality. Concentrate on your breathing, allowing it to involve the whole of your mind, much as the article you had been taking a gander at did previously. Feel yourself getting progressively loose with each extra breath.

Envision that the entirety of the strain and stress are disseminating from your muscles. Permit this inclination to descend your body from your face, to your chest, your arms, lastly, your legs.

When you are loosened up, your mind should be clear, and you will be part way to self-hypnosis.

5. **Envision a pendulum**. The movement of a swing moving back and forward has generally been utilized in hypnosis to support the center. In your mind, envision this pendulum moving back and forward. Concentrate on it as you unwind to help clear your mind.

6. **Tally down to hypnosis**. Start including down in your mind from 10 to 1. As you tally down, disclose to yourself that you are getting dynamically more profound into hypnosis. State, "10, I am unwinding. 9. I am getting progressively loose. 8, I can feel the unwinding spreading down my body. 7, I can feel only the unwinding 1, I am in a profound rest."

Recall all through that when you arrive at 1, you will be in a condition of hypnosis.

7. **Wake up**. When you have achieved what you need during hypnosis, you should wake yourself. Tally back up from 1 to 10. In your mind, say: "1, I am awakening: 2, when I tally down, I will feel like I woke from a profound rest. 3, I am feeling progressively alert 10, I am alert and invigorated."

Section 2. Persuading Yourself to Lose Weight While Under Hypnosis

1. **Build up a routine**. It takes reliable reiteration to

reconstruct your mind with hypnosis. You should expect to go through around twenty minutes per day in a condition of hypnosis. While under, switch back and forth between a portion of the procedures recorded beneath. Attempt a touch of everything to assault your terrible dietary patterns from each point accessible.

2. **Figure out how to detest undesirable foods**. One of the main things you should attempt to do while under hypnosis is to persuade yourself that you aren't keen on the frightful nibble foods that you're experiencing difficulty kicking. Pick something like frozen yogurt that you will, in general, revel in. Let yourself know, "Frozen yogurt tastes awful and causes me to feel wiped out." Repeat for twenty minutes, until you are prepared to alert from hypnosis.

Keep in mind; a decent diet doesn't imply that you have to quit eating; simply eat less terrible foods. Try not to convince yourself not to eat; simply to persuade yourself to eat less food that you know is unfortunate.

3. **Compose your own positive mantra**. You ought to likewise utilize self-hypnosis to strengthen your longing to eat better. Compose a mantra that to rehash while in a condition of hypnosis. Models include: "Overeating harms me and my body. I ought to eat beneficial to make myself a superior me."

4. **Envision a superior you**. To increase your longing to live better, imagine what you would resemble sound.

Snap a photo of yourself from when you were more slender or put forth a valiant effort to envision what you would resemble in the wake of losing weight. Under hypnosis, center around this picture. Envision the certainty that you would feel if you were more advantageous. This will make you need to understand that more slender you when you wakeful.

Section 3. Keeping up a Healthy Diet

1. **Eat protein with each supper**. Protein is particularly acceptable at topping you off and, because it bolsters muscle development, can really improve your digestion. Great wellsprings of protein incorporate seafood, lean meat, eggs, yogurt, nuts, and beans. A steak each supper may be counterproductive. However, eating on nuts when you're ravenous could help you reach your objectives.

2. **Eat a few small suppers a day**. At the point when you don't eat for an all-inclusive timeframe, your digestion goes down, and you quit burning fat. If you eat something small once every three or four hours, your digestion will go up, and you will be less eager when you plunk down for dinner.

3. **Eat products of the soil**. Foods grown from the ground will top you off and flexibly you with supplements without putting any pounds on. Nibble on

bananas rather than treats to begin losing weight.

4. **Cut down on awful fats**. Unsaturated fats, similar to those in olive oil, can be beneficial for you. You should, in any case, attempt to confine your utilization of soaked fats and trans fats. Both of these are significant contributing variables in coronary illness.

Trans fats are healthy in prepared foods, especially heated products, icing, and margarine.

Soaked fats are not as awful as trans fats, but they can be undesirable. Significant wellsprings of saturated fat incorporate margarine, cheddar, fat, red meat, and milk.

Weight loss made easy

With regards to losing weight, you definitely think about the standard go-to professionals: specialists, nutritionists, and dietitians, fitness coaches, even psychological well-being mentors. Be that as it may, there might be the one you haven't precisely thought of yet: a trance specialist.

It turns out utilizing hypnosis is another street people are wandering down for the sake of weight loss. Regularly, it's gone after the various final desperate attempts (I see you, juice scrubs, and craze diets) are attempted and fizzled.

Be that as it may, it's not about another person controlling your mind and causing you to do exciting things while you're oblivious. "Mind control and losing control—otherwise known as accomplishing something against your will—are the greatest misguided judgments about hypnosis. Because of how media outlets depict trance inducers, people are calmed to see I'm not wearing a dark robe and swinging a watch from a chain."

You're likewise not oblivious when you experience hypnosis—it's progressively similar to a covert government of unwinding. "It's just the characteristic, floaty inclination you get before you drift off to rest or that marvelous sensation you feel as you get up in the first part of the prior day you're completely mindful of where you are and what is encompassing you."

Being in that state makes you progressively defenseless to change, which is why hypnosis for weight loss might be successful. "It's different from different techniques because hypnosis tends to the reason and other contributing elements straightforwardly at the subconscious level in the individual's mind, where their recollections, propensities, fears, food affiliations, negative self-talk, and confidence grow. No other weight loss strategy tends to the central issues at the root as hypnosis does."

But, does hypnosis for weight loss work?

There isn't a huge amount of later, randomized

examination accessible regarding the matter, yet what is out there recommends that the strategy could be conceivable. Early examinations from the 90s found that people who utilized hypnosis lost more than twice as much weight as the individuals who dieted without subjective treatment. A 2014 study worked with 60 corpulent ladies and found that the individuals who rehearsed Hypno-conduct treatment shed pounds and improved their dietary patterns and body picture. What's more, a small 2017 study worked with eight stout grown-ups and three youngsters, every one of whom effectively shed pounds, with one, in any event, staying away from the medical procedure because of the treatment benefits, none of this is definitive.

"The awful factor is that hypnosis isn't promptly secured by clinical protection, so there isn't a similar push for hypnosis reads as there is for pharmaceutical ones."

Who should attempt hypnosis for weight loss?

The perfect applicant is, truly, any individual who experiences difficulty adhering to a solid diet and exercise program because they can't shake their negative propensities. Stalling out in destructive propensities— like eating the whole sack of potato chips as opposed to halting when you're full—is an indication of a subconscious issue.

Your subconscious is the place your feelings,

propensities, and addictions are found. Furthermore, because hypnotherapy addresses the subconscious— rather than simply the conscious—it might be increasingly powerful. Indeed, a study investigation from 1970 discovered hypnosis to have a 93 percent achievement rate, with fewer meetings required than both psychotherapy and social treatment. "This persuaded, for evolving propensities, thought examples, and conduct, hypnosis was the best technique."

Hypnotherapy doesn't need to be utilized all alone, either. Hypnosis can likewise be utilized as a commendation to other weight loss programs structured by professionals to treat different wellbeing conditions, be it diabetes, stoutness, joint inflammation, or cardiovascular malady.

What would I be able to expect during a treatment?

Meetings can change long and system relying upon the specialist. As a rule, you can hope to set down, unwind with your eyes closed, and let the subliminal specialist control you through specific strategies and suggestions that can assist you with arriving at your objectives.

"The thought is to prepare the mind to advance toward what is solid and away based on what is unfortunate. Through customer history, I am ready to decide subconscious hitches that sent the customer off their unique diagram of [health]. Much the same as we figure out how to mishandle our bodies with food, we can figure out how to respect them."

What's more, no, you won't cackle like a chicken or admitting any profound, dull privileged insights. "You can't be stuck in hypnosis or made to state or accomplish something against your will. If it conflicts with your own qualities or convictions, you essentially won't follow up on the data being given during stupor."

Instead, almost certainly, you'll experience a profound unwinding while still monitoring what's being said. "Somebody in an entrancing stupor would portray it as in the middle of being wide conscious and sleeping. They are completely in charge and ready to stop the procedure whenever, because you must be spellbound if you decide to. We fill in as a group to accomplish the individual's objective."

The quantity of meetings required is absolutely subject to your own reaction to hypnosis. Some could get results in as not many as one to three, while others could require somewhere in the range of eight to 15 meetings. And afterward again, it may not be successful for everybody.

CHAPTER FOUR: STEP BY STEP HYPNOTHERAPY FOR WEIGHT LOSS

You are baffled for not fitting into your last year's garments. Bouncing to greater sizes is making you strained. You no more end up glancing in the mirror because you are apprehensive.

You have skirted a couple of social functions of late and are attempting your best to confine yourself.

At a cognizant level, you know about all the reasons why you ought to lose weight. You genuinely wish to dispose of all the additional rotundity and get back fit as a fiddle. You have tried each supernatural occurrence pill, attempted each extravagant diet plan, and exercised vigorously in the rec center; however, it fizzled.

Thus, you are currently miserable, disheartened, and discouraged.

Intentionally, you are persuaded to begin eating well and exercise routinely, yet somewhere inside, there lies an amazing power that urges you to put off every single sound conduct inevitably.

Have you asked why?

This is because your subconscious mind is shielding you from "losing" anything. This may appear to be another plan for you, yet it is exceptionally evident.

Your subconscious is resolved to shield you from losing your expectation, your way, your rest, your cash, and your time. It's frustrating that your subconscious mind will go to any length to shield you from losing weight as well.

This default lies somewhere down in your cognizant mind, and regardless of how solid your cognizant endeavors are, it continues interfering in your weight loss objective.

Things being what they are, is that it? Will you always be unable to lose weight?

Obviously, not.

"Your subconscious is normally modified to shield you from losing your expectation, your way, your rest, your cash, and even your body weight."

Self-hypnosis for weight loss may be another idea for you, yet it is being used for quite a while. By utilizing this procedure, you re-program your subconscious mind to allow your body to discharge the additional pounds.

Subsequently, your mind changes your metabolic rate, craving, and physical vitality by means of neurohormones, just to quicken weight loss.

Utilizing self-hypnosis for weight loss can help you change the way you take a gander at exercise, food, and even yourself. You will, in general, beginning carrying on as a thin individual, and it comes all normally.

Along these lines, disregard obsessing about calories and constraining yourself to the rec center. Follow these six straightforward strides to utilize self-hypnosis for weight loss now.

Stage 1

Discover time in your day when any external components do not divert you. Put aside at any rate 30 minutes to drench yourself in a daze. It is critical to stay centered during this timeframe.

Stage 2

Set a weight-loss focus for yourself. Focus on an accurate measure of weight you wish to lose and the specific time frame for it. Make sure to peruse this objective out loud before starting.

Stage 3

Begin envisioning yourself as the size you want to

accomplish. Envision how your body will look like once you have achieved your optimal weight. Consider what others will say about your changed looks. Attempt to picture the scene as strikingly as possible under the circumstances, with vibrant hues, sounds, scents, and emotions.

Stage 4

Close your eyes, and have a go at loosening up your body until it releases. Watch deep breathing for around three minutes until you feel a sensation moving from your skull right to your feet. When the sensation is felt, take a stab at loosening up that piece of the body. This will assist you in getting into an unconscious state.

Stage 5

Presently, envision your ideal self in a state of stupor. Consider your point of view with respect to the world, how others will respond, and how good you will feel to be in extraordinary shape. Watch your body in its trim state.

Stage 6

Continuously come back to your current state. Guarantee that you carry the sentiments of internal involvement in you on your way back. Rehash it consistently to prepare your mind about how good it will be to dispose of the weight. Before long, you will wind up making conduct modifications essential to losing fat.

Try not to expect that self-hypnosis may cause you to do things you don't plan to. It can't. Indeed, it will assist you with arriving at your weight loss goals. Recall that it is you who is always in control.

CHAPTER FIVE: 1 HOUR GUIDED MEDITATION HYPNOSIS TO ASSIST YOU WITH LOSING WEIGHT AND EAT HEALTHILY

Reasons why meditation is helpful in weight loss

Is it accurate to say that you are losing rest in your endeavors to lose weight? Hasn't exercise helped you reduce body weight as much as you had trusted? Do fatty food things shout to you despite your most steadfast dismissals?! Never dread, meditation is here!

Accomplish you tenaciously work out at the exercise center for extended periods? Have you additionally prepared your taste buds to prefer servings of mixed greens over seared bites? If you have, without a doubt, the gauging machine is mixed up? Such discipline thus little to appear for it! What more would you be able to do? All things considered, what about adding something familiar and easy to your day by day schedule? Have you attempted meditation to lose weight?

Is it true that you are thinking about how this is even

identified with weight loss? Meditation is for the mind, not the body, right? Indeed, if you consider it, losing weight is as much a psychological procedure as a physical one. If you could prepare your mind to deny lousy nourishment, you have won half the fight.

In this way, we should investigate what meditation can accomplish for weight loss:

Meditation tips for weight loss

1. Meditation lowers your BMR easily

What number of calories do you need very still? Just to continue breathing. That is your BMR or Basal Metabolic Rate. So the lower, the better. Lower calorie-intake implies reduced body weight. Sufficiently basic. In any case, how? At the point when you ponder, your body's BMR reduces. This implies you need fewer calories, and this causes you to lose weight - normally.

2. Meditation helps in the digestion of food

All in all, you worked out at the exercise center for 60 minutes? You should be eager. You believe you could eat quite a bit after a thorough exercise routine. What's more, you nearly do! Nonetheless, the upsetting truth is that your increased craving proceeds in any event, when you don't work out. The issue emerges with the absorption of the food you expend. How might you improve that to lose weight?

Indeed, perhaps the best tip for weight loss is to practice meditation. Meditation improves the digestion of food. Hormonal awkwardness and stress lead to gorging and heartburn. It loosens up your focus on nerves and parity your hormones. This has a drawn-out impact on your endeavors at weight loss. Thus, regardless of whether you don't exercise for a couple of days, you won't gain a lot of weight.

3. Meditation moderates unhealthy inclinations for cheap food

The greatest detour to weight loss is, maybe, wanting for low-quality nourishment, particularly if you have a sweet tooth or are a foodie. What meditation can accomplish for you is to make you increasingly mindful. At the point when you are in the 'mindfulness zone,' it is simpler to dismiss those scrumptious allurements. You become progressively careful about what you eat. After some time, your yearnings for those mouth-watering cakes and chips will likewise reduce.

4. Meditation = Less pressure

Have you watched precisely when you go after that pack of chips or that bar of chocolate? Is it safe to say that you were worried at that point and searching for some speedy 'innocuous' thrills? You may not always feel it; however, stress can situate itself deeply in your system. It prompts over guilty pleasures. This is the reason meditation is so successful for weight loss. It alleviates your burden by connecting to your internal identity and discharging you of your weights. At the point when you are loose, you won't have any desire to attack the larder.

5. Meditation boosts duty

Day 1 and Day 10 of your weight-loss program are, presumably, the hardest. Taking off requires activity, however keeping up the routine is no bit of cake either! You need the pledge to proceed. Despite your best goals, there are dangers. For example, resting excessively or excessively little, and devouring inexpensive food. These upset your weight loss program by debilitating your resolve.

Meditation invigorates you the determination and to understand your expectation. You figure out how to esteem your responsibility to exercise by following a moderate diet. Thus, practice meditation consistently to lose weight.

6. You have no time to exercise

Have you at any point revealed to yourself this? Get this: meditation will assist you with discovering additional time during the day!

"I have such a great amount to achieve today that I should ruminate for two hours instead of one."

Meditation makes you progressively effective, giving you the inclination that you were gifted additional time. It will assist you in setting aside a few minutes for exercise.

Before you practice meditation for weight loss, you could do some yoga asanas. Diet is additionally a crucial piece of each weight loss program, and these tips for weight loss can work ponders.

Toward the day's end, figure out how to acknowledge and love yourself as you seem to be. Sometimes, when you drop your mind weight loss, you begin to lose weight!

We should burn a couple of pounds of those annoying pounds off with this yoga workout for weight loss! Yoga is an unfathomable type of exercise that can be utilized for adaptability, strength, and, indeed, losing weight.

It profoundly affects weight loss, and this workout will help burn off belly fat quicker than any time in recent memory!

This yoga workout for weight loss will likewise help with vitality levels and adaptability, giving the body a restored feeling of purpose and the additional vitality to burn more calories.

Who is the workout for?

Vessel Pose (Navasana)

Vessel Posture - Navasana is outstanding amongst other

yoga poses for weight loss.

Gradually raise your legs up to a 45-degree edge, utilizing your arms to enable you to adjust. When you feel adjusted and steady enough, gradually raise your arms to the outside of the knees.

Hold for 30 seconds. Work towards holding this situation for an entire moment.

Plank Pose (Phalakasana)

Solidly grasp the mat, round the shoulders and upper back, and keep your butt in line with the remainder of your body. Try not to let your body hang by any stretch of the imagination. Remain firm and tight, and the abs will accomplish all the work for you!

Hold for 30 seconds. Work up to holding it for 2 minutes.

Bridge Variation (Setu Bandha Sarvangasana)

Bridge Variation is an incredible pose for weight loss.

Start by laying flat on the ground with your knees bowed and heels contacting your butt. Utilize your glutes and center to lift yourself up and balance on the feet and shoulders.

Arrive at your arms underneath you and alter your shoulders so that you can raise yourself higher.

Gradually lift up your right leg and hold. Ensure your left knee is at a 90-degree point.

Hold for 30 seconds. Perform on the two sides.

Side Plank Variation (Vasisthasana)

Start in side plank pose with your left hand on the mat directly beneath your left shoulder and your feet at an edge. Gradually arrive at your right leg up to your right arm. Get your toes if you can while keeping the right leg straight.

This requires a great deal of adaptability in the legs. If you can't straighten the leg, have a go at twisting your knee somewhat.

Superman Pose (Viparita Shalabhasana)

Delicately raise your head, chest, arms, and feet up simultaneously. Your lower belly and hips ought to stay flat on the ground. Raise them up as high as possible and hold. Your look ought to be straight in front of you.

Hold for 30 seconds. Attempt to work up to holding it for as long as 1 moment.

If you are worn out on feeling substantial and in torment from your additional weight and are keen on losing weight rapidly with a calm yoga practice, try to investigate our Yoga Fat Loss Bible for Beginners!

Upward (Reverse) Plank Pose (Purvottanasana)

Start in the passing on position with your legs before you and your hands put directly underneath your shoulders. Utilizing your center and your glutes, lift your body up until your pelvis is directly in a straight line with the remainder of your body.

Hold this situation for 30 seconds.

Half Moon Pose (Ardha Candrāsana)

Half Moon Pose - Ardha Candrāsana is an extraordinary yoga poses to assist you with losing weight.

Attempt to stack the hips with the goal that the body is open and pointing outwards, not down towards the mat.

Point your right foot out to the side also, not the floor. If you don't have the adaptability to arrive at the floor while keeping your left leg straight, twist the left knee marginally to permit your hand to contact the floor (or utilize a yoga square).

Different modifications incorporate arriving at your right arm towards the floor to help with parity or arriving at your left arm to your knee instead of the floor.

Hold for 30 seconds. Perform on the two sides.

Side Plank Variation (Vasisthasana)

Start in side plank pose with your right hand on the mat directly beneath your right shoulder and your feet at a point. Gradually arrive at your right leg around and before your right leg. Curve the knee with the goal that it's at a 90-degree edge.

Arrive at your left arm towards the roof, and let your look lift upward.

Hold for 30 seconds. Perform on the two sides.

Side Angle Pose (Utthita Parsvakonasana)

Start in Warrior I (a thrust position with your left knee bowed forward at a 90-degree edge, and your right leg straight back with your toes pointed forward). Twist the left elbow and let it lay on the right knee (or arrive at it to the cold earth to increase the stretch). Arrive at your right arm up behind you, so it's in a straight line with your right leg.

Increase the stretch in your side body by connecting farther through your right fingertips.

Hold for 30 seconds. Rehash on the two sides.

Four-Limbed Staff Pose (Chaturanga Dandasana)

This is a plank variation. Chaturanga is additionally the yogi push-up.

From the plank position, lower your whole body until your middle corresponds to your upper arms and triceps. Ensure that your butt is lifted somewhat higher than your center and that your belly isn't drooping. Remain firm.

To start with, have a go at holding this situation for 10 seconds. Work up 30 seconds – 1 moment.

Wheel Pose (Chakrasana)

This is a further developed pose (contingent upon your common back adaptability); however, we needed to add it in here to help challenge you!

Start by laying flat on your back with your knees bowed and your heels contacting your butt. Twist your elbows, and spot your palms face down on either side of your head. Delicately propel yourself up, utilizing your arms and your feet.

Be mindful of the elbows. They will, in general, need to stand out in this position.

Hold it for 30 seconds or as long as you feel great.

Crow Pose (Bakasana)

This pose is somewhat more progressed, yet it has been incorporated to assist you with testing yourself.

Start in a hunching down situation behind you with your hands out before you. Come up onto your toes, and spot your knees on your upper arms, as close to your armpits as could reasonably be expected. Gradually shift your weight forward until your feet fall off of the ground and your arms are supporting your weight.

To modify this for novices, have a go at putting your knees closer to your elbows or even only outside of your elbows.

Hold for 30 seconds or as long as could be expected under the circumstances.

Recall that for this workout, you will hold each pose for 30 seconds before moving onto the following pose. After every one of the 12 poses has been finished, rest for one moment.

At that point, rehash the workout, doing sure to turn sides on the poses that work different sides of the body. Rest for an extra moment, and complete the poses for the third time.

Don't hesitate to remain in any of the stretches for longer than 30 seconds if it feels good on your body or you think you need it.

CHAPTER SIX: FAT BURNING ACTIVATION WITH HYPNOSIS

To lose weight, it's significant that your digestion is in top working request because that is what is answerable for burning the fat in your body.

So to cause your body to burn increasingly fat, there are a few things you can do to drive your digestion into high rigging.

1. Exercise before anything else

You aren't as worn out as you would be in the wake of a monotonous day. Also, it is a lot simpler to think of reasons not to exercise toward the day's end.

Practicing toward the beginning of the day gets your digestion wrenching first thing, and this will assist it with remaining dynamic during the entire day.

If practicing at night is the main alternative for you, this is still extremely helpful. You can see here for the science behind when really to exercise.

2. Get into the cardio mode

Ways to burn fat

You have to get your heart siphoning with the goal of taking your body to a level where it burns fat. This implies you have to escape your usual range of familiarity a piece, as it is commonly a point where you are exhausted and getting a sweat on.

Attempt a walk/run, a wellness class, a lively swim meeting, the cardio meetings from Exercise DVD, or some cycling.

3. Weights and quality training

Having more muscle in your body implies you can burn fat all the more proficiently – it can likewise boost your digestion!

So doing some quality training (sit-ups, push-ups, the plank) and a few weights (hand weights can even be a tin of beans) can be extremely valuable for getting progressively conditioned and losing fat.

4. Appreciate good fats, healthy carbs, and quality proteins

It's critical to get the right blend of supplements from the entirety of the food gatherings – which is the reason we never suggest removing certain foods from your diet.

Attempt to get the blend of fat/carb/protein in every supper – for example, breakfast may be avocado, wholegrain toast, and a poached egg.

5. Try not to skip suppers or go hungry

The body needs food for fuel. If it doesn't get it, it goes into starvation mode (AKA fat stockpiling mode), which is the specific inverse of where we need to be.

Try not to get so hungry that your feelings assume control over your sane mind and eat unhealthy foods.

Plan ahead with the goal of having your dinners and bites all set, so you aren't enticed to avoid a supper when you're occupied or purchase low-quality nourishment when you're all over town.

The Healthy Mummy Smoothies are an incredible way to begin the day if you find that your mornings are occupied and unpleasant!

6. Express yes to flavor

Bean stew and hot food is a delicious way to get your digestion turning. It is as straightforward as including slashed bean stew or even jalapenos to a portion of your dinners every week.

7. Top off on fiber

Fiber gets your stomach related system fit as a fiddle and assists with freeing the body of waste. Did you realize that each service of the Healthy Mummy Smoothie contains 6g of fiber? Furthermore, that is before you include any milk, natural product, or veggies.

You can likewise discover fiber in natural products, for example, raspberries, oranges, apples, pears, and mango; herbs and flavors like cinnamon, thyme, cloves, rosemary and coriander; and in nuts and seeds as well.

8) Drink a lot of water

Each system in the body needs water to function, including your digestion. So make it simple on your body by toting around your water bottle and tasting normally, so you don't get dried out.

The most effective method to ACTIVATE YOUR FAT-BURNING GENE

Presently we will talk about the good sort of fat, brown fat. It's classified "good" fat because it burns calories and discharges vitality, in contrast to "terrible" white fat that basically stores additional calories.

Brown fat is composed of countless iron-containing

mitochondria (the cell's warmth burning motor), which is the thing that gives the brownish appearance (white fat needs mitochondria).

The purpose of brown fat is to burn calories so as to produce heat. That is why brown fat is referred to as "good" fat, causing us to burn, not store calories.

"Only 50 grams of brown fat in one's body can burn up 20% of a person's day by day caloric intake. It's essentially a fire that is persistently burning vitality (calories) in the body."

People who have increasingly brown fat will, in general, be leaner, more advantageous, and have ordinary blood sugar levels.

Along these lines, try to enact your "fat-burning qualities" to produce and trigger this brown fat and let the body burn away the vitality put away in its abundance white fat. You're molding your body to be a productive fat-burner 24 hours per day, seven days every week. Here are a few of your fat-burning qualities:

Your Fat Burning Genes

PRDM16

PRDM16 (PR area containing 16) is a fat-burning quality got from protein that fills in as the "ace controller" of brown fat turn of events. It really changes over cells from white fat into calorie-burning brown fat.

Analysts found that when the PRDM16 quality was expelled from brown fat, the cells quit being metabolic powerhouses and were really transformed into white fat.

Ucp1

Brown fat contains another fat-burning quality called Ucp1 (uncoupling protein 1), and when enacted, it burns off fat to produce heat, a procedure called "thermogenesis."

The principle weight loss advantage of thermogenesis is that it goes through putting away vitality (white fat). For our body to create heat, it needs to burn calories. Furthermore, since these calories originate from our body fat stores, we clearly need to trigger, however much thermogenesis as could be expected.

The Ucp1 works in the mitochondria of the brown ("good") fat to deliver ATP, which utilizes that fuel to make heat and, in this way, burn fat. Here's only one way to trigger this.

The foods you eat can cause or increase thermogenesis, and this way, your "calorie burn rate." Foods wealthy in lean protein cause the greatest increase in thermogenesis. Certain carbs additionally make thermogenesis, particularly when joined with the right sorts of protein.

Along these lines, try to join the right sort of protein and certain carbs together to make thermogenesis, which can make a 10 to 15% everyday calorie use. In this way, if you expended 2.500 calories every day, this would make an interpretation from 250 to 375 additional calories burned every day - just by eating the right sorts of food together.

Here are probably the best thermogenesis-instigating foods:

Flavors: devouring foods with flavors, for example, intensely hot peppers or dark pepper, increases thermogenesis and can significantly affect sentiments of satiety and fat oxidation. Capsaicin, the substance that gives spicy peppers their impactful flavor, has been accounted for to increase thermogenesis. Correspondingly, dark pepper contains piperine, a substance that has appeared to impact thermogenesis through animating the sensory system.

Green tea: contains two substances - caffeine and polyphenols called catechins - that have appeared to boost thermogenesis and may upgrade each other's belongings. Catechins in green tea may increase thermogenesis by repressing a specific protein. Green tea contains high-level measures of specific catechin called epigallocatechin gallate, which is likely the most pharmacological dynamic.

Coconut oil: contains predominantly medium-chain fatty acids - fats that, when devoured, have been appeared to hinder fat affidavit through increased thermogenesis and fat burning, in considers led in creatures and people.

Proteins: are the most thermogenic food, including lean meat, poultry, eggs, fish and shellfish, curds, Greek yogurt, protein powder, and nuts.

At the point when you join lean proteins with fundamental "healthy" fats, just as sinewy carbs (vegetables), your body will actually transform into a fat-burning machine. Here's a straightforward 3-advance recipe to assemble a fat-burning feast.

Stage 1: Select a stringy carb (vegetable high in fiber, for example, broccoli, asparagus, green beans, brussel grows, cauliflower, spinach, kale, and so forth, and afterward.)

Stage 2: Combine it with a high lean protein (lean meat, fish, or low-fat dairy).

Stage 3: The lean protein and stringy carb structures the establishment of your fat-burning dinner - and is excellent if later in the day. In any case, if it's prior in the day when your body needs more vitality, you'll need to include a characteristic dull carb, for example, brown rice, oats, potatoes, sweet potatoes, or yams. Straightforward carbs (organic product) prior in the day (or after a workout), straightforward carbs (organic product) work well.

Outline: you can turn on qualities that make weight loss

simpler by actuating brown fat.

CHAPTER SEVEN: HEAL YOUR RELATIONSHIP WITH FOOD

Negative sentiments about food and weight can crash even the most beneficial of lifestyles. If you have a loaded relationship with specific foods or a background marked by enthusiastic dieting or pigging, here are a few methodologies that can help you begin to break the cycle:

1. Quit rebuffing yourself for what you ate yesterday

Choosing not to move on doesn't serve you or your body. Everything it does is cause pressure and tension—which just drives you further from wellbeing and bliss.

2. Practice mindful eating

Plunk down and draw in your faculties with each dinner: Smell food, take a gander at it and taste it with appreciation. Make an effort not to work on your PC or read as you're eating. Instead, dedicate all your thoughtfulness to what's on your plate. This can assist you with eating slower and better review your food.

3. Have an appreciation for your food

Stop and consider how this food got to your plate and that you are so fortunate to approach it. It is a gift that is going to feed your body.

4. Permit yourself to make the most of your food

If negative contemplations like, "I ought not to be eating this" or "I'm a disappointment that I was unable to control what I ate" emerge as you're eating, permit them to go without judgment. At that point, return to appreciation.

5. Stop horrendous win or bust cycles

Numerous people will eat a donut and afterward think, "Well, since I previously ate garbage, I should simply prop up for the entire [day, end of the week, etc.]." Thinking like this can prompt a food gorge that closes in blame and disgrace. Recall that one food decision doesn't have to direct the following.

6. Practice positive affirmations

Positive affirmations are a useful asset for switching negative considerations and acting in arrangement with your qualities. Here are some that have helped me improve my relationship with food throughout the years:

- This plate of food is so good for me.
- My body realizes how to utilize this food.
- My body and soul are going to be supported with so much goodness.

7. Relinquish should be great

Nobody eats "consummately" since impeccable doesn't exist. Attempt to discharge the requirement for flawlessness by recollecting that you are actually where you should be.

8. Quit contrasting your plate with other people's

You have different dietary needs than your companions, family, and associates. Their relationship with food has nothing to do with you.

9. Try not to let a healthy lifestyle hinder your public activity

If you're out with loved ones, don't pressure if the food alternatives aren't the most advantageous. Necessarily pick the most engaging thing accessible to you in that circumstance. Recall that remunerating social connections are a structure square of wellbeing, as well, similarly as nutritious food may be.

10. If you're going after food when you're not ravenous, ask yourself how you're feeling inwardly

For what reason would you say you are going after solace as food? Might you be able to discover it somewhere else? Consider taking a stroll outside, cleaning up, or calling up a companion instead.

11. Recollect this is your one body

Fortune it. Take care of it. Fill it with supplements. Express gratitude toward it for all that it accomplishes for you, every day.

CHAPTER EIGHT: HEALING THE BODY WITH HYPNOSIS

The right food, proper exercise, the right prescriptions, and the right connections can bolster your mending procedure, however, not unless you deliberately prompt them. Your cognizant, purposeful mind (which is independent of, however, associated with, your inner mind and sensory system) is simply the way to your recuperating.

The procedure is straightforward.

To start with, you have to comprehend the procedure with your astuteness, the part fit for basic reasoning that understands the estimation of proof-based thinking.

The subsequent stage in mending any system is that the system gets mindful of its way of life as a system. For you, this implies liberating yourself from interruption and concentrating on what your identity is, your actual qualities, purpose, goals, and vision.

Third, you figure out how to peruse the signs and messages that originate from within and how to adjust your system — truly, mentally, and inwardly.

Luckily, you can figure out how to do this in an amazingly brief timeframe utilizing the ground-breaking Mind Tools. These devices can help you reach a wonderful state of deep relaxation and meditation, carrying you into the present, discharging your mind of interruptions and your body of poisons, and setting up the cells of your body to get your self-mending directions.

Another entirely important instrument for self-recuperating is guided imagery. This procedure includes holding specific mending imagery in the mind while in the responsive "Recuperating State." This results in the help of pressure, and the enactment of your oblivious recuperating and restorative procedures are prepared. Undeniably, you are "reprogramming" your mind and revamping your cerebrum. You will probably restore internal coherence and parity, and along these lines to help mend your body, feelings, mind, and conduct.

Each time you rehash these encounters, you are re-scripting your body, your passionate state, and how you will react in future circumstances. You will find this is an amazing way to rehearse mentally, through guided imagery, your ideal practices of mind and body, much as competitors or actors mentally rehearse their exhibitions.

These new practices may have to do with modifying how the internal organs of your body work, how you converse with yourself, your personal habits, how you connect with others, and so on. Diet, exercise, rest, petition, meditation, and different modalities of re-adjusting the system might be required; however, all these expect us to change our psychological conduct so as to apply them. In this way, the mind-body pivot is always essential in recuperating yourself. Change Your Mind – Change Your Life.

Relaxation — Deep Relaxation is fundamental for fast recuperating because it is the immediate antitoxin to push. Likewise, relaxation exhausts your mind of interruptions, and in this way permits you to self-program new, increasingly alluring self-recuperating practices — both at the obvious (naturally visible) level and in the minuscule conduct of the phones of your body. Deep relaxation is likewise the way to programming mind and body for top execution in any undertaking — sports, profession, or personal life (truly, even sexual).

Entering "The Healing State" — Here, the mind is available to re-scripting, and the body acknowledges new healthy pictures and feelings. Re-scripting is a ground-breaking way to mentally rehearse wanted practices of the mind and body, much as competitors or actors mentally rehearse their exhibitions. These guided imagery and meditation CDs and MP3 downloads will teach you to do this through basic, intelligent, straightforward, and exceptionally pleasant guided imagery encounters. The experience and your capacity to utilize the Healing State turns out to be logically increasingly amazing with a couple of moments a day of pleasurable practice.

Framing Powerful, Transformative, Healing Images — Intentional mental imagery through Selective Awareness — Software For The Mind — permits you to make a guarantee to mending yourself by directly affecting the conduct of the cells of your body (e.g., the safe system), starting and continuing wellbeing delivering practices, (exercise, diet, non-maltreatment of liquor or medications, quit smoking), and produce wellbeing supporting self-picture. This inward picture serves to change the conduct at each degree of the mind-body system.

Practicing These Images Daily — Reprogramming your mind is really retraining the mind. Similarly, as you would practice melodic scales or composing so as to improve, the ordinary practice of the fitting imagery prepares the mind, the sensory system, and the resistant system to do the ideal changes effectively. You will probably restore internal coherence and equalization and along these lines to help recuperate the body, feelings, mind, and conduct.

Strengthening Positive Changes — Reward your mind for reacting to your pleas with the goal that the new practices win. Take yourself out for supper, to a ball game, or a film, for example. Or then again, go on vacation to be with loved ones.

CHAPTER NINE: DAILY WEIGHT LOSS MOTIVATION WITH MINI HABITS

Neither 30-day diets nor 10-day juice fasts are genuine answers for weight loss. These are outside conduct and dietary abnormalities that your mind and body will compel right in time. They can make the dream of change, yet unless your mind's neural pathways change through maintainable reiteration, you will return to who you, despite everything, are underneath.

It's no riddle why craze diets and "cleanses" get famous. People get fast, brief outcomes, which energizes them enough to tell everybody they know. Long haul, their prosperity isn't continued—they recover the weight—however, the makers of these transient plans just need that underlying energy to make their business soar.

The Only Permanent Solution

The main perpetual weight loss arrangement originates from a lasting change in the person. That is something that no diet has had the option to accomplish with consistency. Nor should we anticipate that they should!

Diets are not changing procedures; they're only a recommendation of what food to eat. Most books introducing another diet totally disregard the system and embrace the universal "simply eat along these lines" theory. If endeavored straight up, another diet is an unforgiving, severe change from the standard that is incredibly difficult to keep up after some time.

Calorie checking, the supposed "hostile to diet arrangement," isn't adroitly different than another diet plan. Instead of eating different food than you're utilized to, calorie tallying is eating less food than you're utilized to. It's much to a greater extent a torment, as well, as you need to follow each bit of food you eat and include your calories. I need to solve math problems to kill my alarm clock toward the beginning of the day—I like math—yet I would not have any desire to tally calories!

Who needs to rebuff themselves for life to be more slender? Who needs to micromanage their life to be more slender? Nobody needs to do either; however, they believe it's vital. It's definitely not.

Set up the pieces, and this is the reason such a significant number of people are overweight and feel a feeling of despondency. They consider it to be a decision between being cheerful and getting a charge out of life or weighing less and being more beneficial. With the current writing on weight loss, I totally comprehend the hopelessness. Do you see the difficulty I see?

Most weight loss arrangements don't consider what your identity is right at this point. They just consider about the moves you can make and the impact those activities will have on your body. They leave the genuine change part, the crucial step, up to you. "Check your calories, never eat starches again, lose the dietary fat, and quit eating sugar," they'll state. What's more, you're forgotten about there to figure how to do it. This is the reason long haul diet adherence is so low. An inability to hold fast to something implies that the methodology didn't work.

Any change you endeavor to make ought to be feasible in for all intents and purposes of all conditions. You ought to have the option to do it in the most noticeably terrible tempest of your life. You ought to have the option to do it when you're drained. You ought to have the option to do it when you're unmotivated. What's more, isn't this presence of mind?

Who, while planning to scale a compelling mountain or sail a non-domesticated ocean, packs their rigging with the suspicion of flawless climate? Savvy travelers know to get ready for the most noticeably awful with the goal that they can beat any affliction that may come. For what reason haven't we figured out how to do this with our endeavors to change? At the point when a person doesn't bring snow rigging to a mountain known for snowstorms, we call them silly. At the point when a person expects they will always be persuaded, we cheer for them.

Weightcations

The general purpose of getting to a more advantageous weight is to remain there and experience those advantages. If you arrive and recover your weight later, it's a weightcation.

Would you be able to see an example here?

1. A person receives a diet plan

2. Diet "works" and a person loses weight

3. Person is glad

4. Person drifts back to their ordinary life

5. A person puts on weight and needs to start a better eating routine once more

6. A person gets amped up for another prevailing fashion diet

7. Repeat stage one

The bright side of dieting is contemplating what and the amount you eat. At the point when you're mindful, you're more averse to expend (over the top measures of) unhealthy food and drink. The idea of dieting, in any case, is fundamentally defective.

Weight loss should be an efficient, determined endeavor, not an uncouth race to drop 20 pounds in 20 days or redesign your dietary habits for the time being. The journey to weight loss with mini habits appears to be so unassuming and insignificant from the start. You'll likely begin losing less weight than your companion Nancy, who is on the most recent prevailing fashion smoothie cleanse. It wasn't decent of Nancy to focus on it, either, yet you know Nancy (if your name is Nancy, I implied the other one). Later on, you'll see Nancy's weight loss improvement moderate, stop, and converse as she understands that not eating enough food is somewhat of a bummer.

As Nancy recovers her weight, have you lost some weight; however, you've been surprisingly reliable with your changes. You've appreciated the procedure instead of fearing it, and you don't feel like you're being depleted of life. You're really showing signs of improvement at picking the right foods after some time (such is the enchantment of habits!). A fruitful change methodology will allow you an opportunity and engage you, not limit you, and cause you to feel like a captive to it. At the point when people are confined, they need to getaway. At the point when people are enabled, they can hardly wait to proceed.

Time passes. You've just shed seven pounds, however, you grin, because you didn't do anything outrageous to get those outcomes. Maybe you rolled out small improvements that you realize you can support for the remainder of your life. It's a different inclination. It's not elation as much as it's a developing certainty that not exclusively would you be able to keep on losing weight, yet you can keep it off as long as you need to. You're not only losing weight; you're losing the mindset and habits that bring about weight. You're vanquishing the underlying foundations of weight gain. You're evolving!

Consider it along these lines: In the right condition, a little flash can make a seething inferno. In any case, in another condition, a huge blast may just most recent a second. We will, in general, think the size of the underlying fire matters most, yet it's progressively about what that fire can turn into. Dieting offers a significant blast that rapidly burns out. Mini habits utilize a small fire to fabricate a solid fire that can burn for a lifetime.

The world needs an option in contrast to dieting. It needs Mini Habits for Weight Loss. Abandon dieting for good...

Mental Fitness, Knowledge, and Intelligence

By Quantity

• Read 2 pages in a book

• Read 1 new reality

• Complete one mental exercise or game

• Memorize a gathering of 5-10 words (essential food

item list)

By Time (1 min)

• Attempt to solve a Rubix shape

• Add 1 in addition to 2 (=3); add 3 to that (=6); add 4 to that outcome (=10); etc....

• Spend brief learning another word (upgrade your local language or gain proficiency with an unknown dialect)

Physical Fitness

Exercise mini habits are appropriate for mini mixture habits, which permit you to change over "X times seven days" goals into day by day goals. This is extraordinary for people beginning who need to accomplish something generally difficult, like go to the rec center reliably.

By Quantity

• 1 Push-up

• 1 Sit-up

• 1 Pull-up

• 1 say something every day (gauging yourself increases your mindfulness about your weight and the things that impact it. Because of Marty for this terrific thought. Additionally, how simple is it to step on a scale?)

- Walk/run to the furthest limit of your driveway

- Leave the house at any rate once every day, farther than the letter drop

- Put on your workout clothes (truly)

- Set up your exercise mat, press play on abdominal muscle video, and sit on a mat (you don't need to do the workout, however, cause yourself to do this and you'll likely need to do it at any rate a tad)

- Drive to the rec center (X times every week)

By Time (30 sec)

- Run steps

- Run set up

- Walk

- Dance

- Jumping jacks

- Push-ups

- Sit-ups

- Pull-ups

Wellbeing, Diet, and Well-Being

By Quantity

• Drink one glass of water

• Eat 1 bit of new organic product (natural)

• Eat one serving of new vegetables (natural)

• HYBRID – Eat one serving of mixed greens OR cook one feast at home

• Relax totally once every day (even quickly)

• Stretch 1 body part

• Floss one tooth

• Office workers

• Stand up and move around once consistently at work (delayed sitting is VERY unhealthy)

• Look at something far away for 10 seconds each hour (can join with past)

By Time (1 min)

• Get daylight

• Relax totally

• Stretch

Satisfaction

Therapists have discovered a couple of things that appear to make all people more joyful. They are social associations, being mentally present, thinking positively, focusing on goals, rehearsing gratefulness, giving, and decreasing pressure. Every single Mini Habit makes us more joyful by giving duty and achievement goals, yet here are some specific Mini Habits that should serve to boost your day by day satisfaction considerably more.

Bliss Habits Warning: Habits are less passionate ordinarily. This implies if you build up the habit of posting three things you're grateful for, the joy impact may wear off as it becomes "schedule." The ideal way to balance this is not to make these things habit purposefully. Instead, you can choose a couple of these and pivot them on every day or week by week premise. This will keep things new and keep you glad and intrigued!

By Quantity

• Write down or consider one thing you're appreciative for

• Write down or ponder life

• Thank one person for something they've accomplished for you

• Say howdy to one outsider

• Connect with one companion

Look at a more unusual (good beginning stage for social improvement)

• Do one thing to reduce your pressure

• Help one person

• Hug one person

• Savor 1 nibble for every dinner

• Smile once (this isn't insignificant)

• Laugh once (grinning/snickering trigger an arrival of feel-good synthetic concoctions in the cerebrum regardless of whether you counterfeit them, however, don't phony them)

By Time (1 min)

• Relax totally or reflect

• Help another person

• Smile/snicker for 10 seconds straight (it makes me giggle simply considering this. Watch these extraordinary laughers if you need a boost—it's infectious!)

Business

By Quantity

• Write down 1 ("lead" for this situation applies to deals or networking)

• Call 1 lead

• Email 1 lead

• Write down 1 business thought

• Ask one client how you can serve them better

• Write down 1 region of your business that could be improved (discretionary: and how to do it)

• Think of 1 new way to streamline your workday (for example, browse email just two times a day)

By Time (1 min)

• Organize paper records

• Organize PC records

• (Re)evaluate your elevated level plan of action

• Brainstorm thoughts (for current or new business)

Profitability

By Quantity

• Plunk a key (on piano, guitar, and so on.)

• "Dejunk" a small surface or region (sink, dresser, 1/2 of work area, bath edge, 3 square feet of floorspace, and so on.)

• Process 1 bit of paper (mail, office docs, and so on.)

• Consume/choose 1 lined thing, (for example, web bookmarks)

• Write 50 words (for a book)

• Write 50 words (for blog)

• Write 50 words (for anything)

• Read 2 pages in a book

• Write three new thoughts

• Learn one new word/state in [language]

By Time (1 min)

• Misc cleaning

• Clean rooms (turn: washroom on Monday, room on Tuesday, and so forth.)

CHAPTER TEN: SELF-HYPNOSIS

Self-hypnosis or auto-hypnosis (as unmistakable from hetero-hypnosis) is a structure, a procedure, or the consequence of a self-prompted trancelike state.

Much of the time, self-hypnosis is utilized as a vehicle to improve the adequacy of self-recommendation, and, in such cases, the subject "assumes the double job of suggester and suggestee."

The idea of the auto-intriguing practice might be, at one extraordinary, "concentrative," wherein all consideration is so completely centered around [the words of the auto-interesting recipe, for example, "Consistently, all around, I'm showing signs of improvement and better"] that everything else is kept out of mindfulness" and, at the other, "comprehensive," wherein subjects "permit a wide range of musings, feelings, recollections, and such to drift into their awareness."

Have you seen old blood and gore movies and TV programs that depict hypnosis as a frightening instrument of mind control where deceitful reprobates oppress the desire of vulnerable casualties? Maybe you have seen stage shows where a trance inducer seems to have the option to utilize their "entrancing forces" to cause people to do and make statements that they could never do or say under typical conditions. If along these lines, it isn't astonishing that hypnosis may appear to be only somewhat wacky, much the same as other apparently magical and unexplainable wonders. This is awful because hypnosis is a genuine restorative device that can assist people with defeating numerous mental, passionate and even some physical problems.

Hypnosis isn't:

• Mind control

• Brain-washing

• Sleep

• Unconsciousness

• A impossible to miss changed state

• A mysterious state

When in hypnosis, a person is:

• Aware

• In control

• In a characteristic and innocuous state

• Able to come out of hypnosis when s/he wishes to

The state of hypnosis can best be depicted as a state of exceptionally engaged consideration with increased suggestibility. Hypnosis is sometimes, however, not always joined by relaxation. At the point when a person, for example, an advisor actuates hypnosis in another, it is called hetero hypnosis, often referred to as hypnotherapy. At the point when hypnosis is self-actuated, it is called autohypnosis and is often referred to as self-hypnosis.

The word hypnosis originates from the Greek word "hypos," which means rest. It is a shortened form of the term neuro-trance induction, which means the rest of the sensory system.

This term was utilized by the prominent neurosurgeon James Braid (1796-1860). Be that as it may, hypnosis isn't a rest state. Indeed, when in hypnosis, a person is conscious and normally mindful of everything that is said and done. Understanding this, Braid later attempted to change the name to monoideaism. This implies a checked distraction with one thought or subject. Be that as it may, the term hypnosis stuck and is utilized right up till the present time.

How Might I Use Self-Hypnosis To Achieve My Goals?

Self-hypnosis is often used to modify conduct, feelings,

and mentalities. For example, numerous people utilize self-hypnosis to help manage the problems of everyday living. Self-hypnosis can boost certainty and even assist people with growing new aptitudes. An extraordinary pressure and tension reliever can likewise be utilized to help defeat habits, for example, smoking and gorging. Athletes can improve their athletic presentation with self-hypnosis, and people experiencing physical agony or stress-related sicknesses also think that its supportive (hypnosis should just be utilized along these lines after a clinical analysis has been done made and under the direction of a specialist or qualified advisor).

A Self-Hypnosis Technique

I will acquaint you with a straightforward, however successful procedure of self-hypnosis. This strategy is called eye obsession self-hypnosis and is one of the most famous and viable types of self-hypnosis at any point created. We will begin by utilizing it as a technique to enable you to unwind. After you have practiced this various times, we will include sleep-inducing proposals and imagery. Reduce interruptions by going into a room where you are probably not going to be upset and killing your telephone, TV, PC, and so forth. This is your time. You are going to concentrate on your objective of self-hypnosis and nothing else.

At that point:

1. Sit in an agreeable seat with your legs and feet uncrossed

Abstain from eating an enormous feast not long previously, so you don't feel enlarged or awkward. Unless you wish to fall asleep, sit in a seat, as resting on a bed will probably prompt rest. You may likewise want to slacken tight clothing and remove your shoes. If you wear contact focal points, it is fitting to expel them. Keep your legs and feet uncrossed.

2. Gaze toward the roof and take in a deep breath

Without straining your neck or inclining your head too far back, pick a point on the roof and fix your look. While you focus your eyes on that point, take a deep breath and hold it for a second and afterward breathe out. Quietly rehash the proposal, "My eyes are worn out and substantial, and I need to SLEEP NOW." Rehash this procedure to yourself another couple of times and, if your eyes have not effectively done as such, let them close and unwind in a normal closed position. It is significant when saying the recommendation that you express it to yourself as though you mean it, for instance, in a delicate, soothing, however persuasive way.

3. Allow your body to unwind

Permit your body to turn out to be free and limp in the seat simply like a cloth doll. At that point, gradually and with goal tally down quietly from five to zero. Disclose to yourself that with every single check, you're turning out to be increasingly loose. Remain in this casual state for several minutes while concentrating on your breathing.

Notice the rising and falling of your stomach and chest. Know how loosened up your body is turning out to be without you in any event, attempting and loosen up it. The less you try, the more loosened up you become.

4. At the point when prepared, return to the room by tallying up from one to five

Reveal to yourself that you are getting mindful of your environmental factors, and at the check of five, you will open your eyes. Check up from one to five of every vivacious, enthusiastic way. At the check of five, open your eyes and stretch your arms and legs.

Rehash this strategy three or four times and notice how each time you arrive at a deeper degree of relaxation. Nonetheless, if you discover you don't unwind as much as you might want, don't compel it. There is an expectation to absorb information included, so resolve to practice self-hypnosis all the time.

Sometimes people will feel somewhat scattered or languid after they come out of the hypnosis. This is like stirring from an evening snooze, is innocuous, and goes after a couple of seconds. Be that as it may, don't drive or work apparatus until you feel completely wakeful.

CHAPTER ELEVEN: HYPNOSIS TRAINING

The accompanying self-hypnosis procedures would all be able to be utilized to make the sleep-inducing state for yourself. They are straightforward yet integral assets that won't just assist you to loosen up deeply and adapt to pressure all the more effectively, but can also assist you with solving problems and conquer personal difficulties. A portion of these will feel higher than others, so it is merely an issue of giving them each of them a shot and discovering one that suits you best. Make self-hypnosis something you do each day, regardless of whether it is for a couple of moments. You don't need to go through hours in deep, devout meditation to feel the advantages. You can do it at set times, or at whatever point the open door emerges, as per your preference and lifestyle. From the outset, utilize these self-hypnosis strategies to unwind and de-stress. This is a significant interest in your prosperity, and will in itself start to assist you with solving problems since you will have more vitality and have the option to think all the more plainly. As you become increasingly acquainted with the different self-hypnosis methods, you can utilize them in a progressively imaginative way, to mentally rehearse a preferred future

– maybe one in which an undesirable habit no longer has an impact, or perhaps envisioning yourself performing great at an approaching occasion, for example, a prospective employee meeting or test. The main necessity for self-hypnosis is comfort and a level of protection, so discover someplace where you can plunk down and stay undisturbed for some time. A force snooze can be exceptionally advantageous; however, it isn't self-hypnosis. A few people additionally prefer to set an alarm clock or timer to keep their self-hypnosis meetings within characterized limits. Once more, this involves personal preference, even though it merits recollecting that we have astoundingly productive body clocks. If you reveal to yourself that you will have fun hypnosis for ten minutes, odds are that you will wind up normally, opening your eyes precisely ten minutes after the fact. Our inner mind continually looks out for us, in any event, when we are sleeping, so if something happens that requires your prompt consideration, you'll be in a split second caution and prepared to manage it. You are probably not going to be so far gone in hypnosis that you don't see the smoke alarm going off. By the by, be reasonable – don't put your deep fat fryer on before settling down and utilizing self-hypnosis!

Three Simple Self Hypnosis Techniques

Every single one of these self-hypnosis procedures works similarly well.

Method 1

Start by concentrating on your breathing. Tune in to your breath and notice how, sooner or later, it starts to back off and deepen of its own agreement. Notice what occurs as you breathe out for longer than you breathe in. Close your eyes at whatever point you feel prepared to do as such. Each time you breathe out, say the word "calm" to yourself in your mind. After a couple of seconds, start to see the word "calm" in your mind's eye as you breathe out. Keep seeing and hearing the word "calm" in your mind, letting it blur away normally as you mentally rehearse your preferred future, or essentially appreciate the deepening vibe of relaxation. At the point when you are prepared to come back to the room, open your eyes.

Method 2

As in the past, start by focusing on your breathing, and permit your eyes to close when you are prepared. As you breathe out, envision an impression of unadulterated relaxation at the highest point of your head. Presently as you breathe out, envision that vibe of relaxation going down from the highest point of your head and over the muscles of your face. Proceed by envisioning that sensation going down into all aspects of your body, from your neck and shoulders, down into your arms, hands, and fingers, and onwards right down to your toes. Rehash twice more, envisioning the sensation growing a little deeper each time. Lead into mental practice or essentially invest some energy simply getting a charge out of the deep relaxation that you have made through the intensity of your creative mind. Tenderly carry yourself to everyday mindfulness by tallying from 1 to 5.

Method 3

As in the past, start by permitting your eyes to close when they're prepared and become mindful of your breathing. Start to develop a psychological picture of a spot where you feel calm, safe, in charge, or positive, and ingenious. This could be a genuine spot, for example, a most loved holiday goal, or it could be absolutely nonexistent. Start by mentally posting all the things you can find in this spot. Proceed onward to investigate the various faculties in this spot – what would you be able to hear, contact, even taste and smell there? As in the past procedures, appreciate this experience for the relaxation that it brings to the table, or use it to lead into sleep-inducing practice.

Self-hypnosis is an instrument to be utilized, instead of a strategy to be fixated on. You would prefer not to be kept down because of an absence of procedure, yet the method isn't the place. Where it's truly at is your main event with what you got." The most significant thing with self-hypnosis is to do it, going with the experience and confiding in it to take you someplace that is totally right and real for you.

CHAPTER TWELVE: SUPER STRAIGHTFORWARD WEIGHT LOSS TIPS

We are given a wide scope of weight loss murmur disperse, the dangers of not getting progressively fit or remaining fit as a fiddle, and so on. Shops and online stores all pass on information on weight loss; weight loss gets inspected all around, restorative centers, working situations, worship houses, and schools. In this way, if you are endeavoring to lose some weight, here are a few hints to fence you on.

Tip 1

Complete just examining weight loss! You won't drop weight by primarily examining it. You've to make a move right now. Here's my suggestion, quit talking and proceed! You'll begin to see a couple of results soon.

Tip 2

Resolute mindsets never lose at long last! A progressive weight loss is better than jumping on some insane diets that never truly work. In case you need to get into shape and keep it off, hope to drop a typical of two pounds step by step. For you to lose some weight, you ought to devour off a bigger number of calories than you take in. Getting exercise together with a diet plan is a prize, diminishing your calorie permit and growing caloric devour rate simultaneously.

Tip 3

Do whatever it takes not to waste your money, don't hurl your merited cash at the latest weight loss trap. Weight loss pills, most new diets, daze, and going under the edge are not the course of action! These things won't meager you down; everyone who advances them essentially removes money from you. Eating right (vegetables, special items, lean proteins, and healthy fats) will help you get more slender faster than the things we get introduced to reliably.

Tip 4

Weight loss is a run of the mill thing. A significant part of us will have weight issues at a couple of centers in our lives. Indulging various took care of sustenances with too little exercise are the two biggest supporters of this steady fight. In case you need to shed pounds and keep it off, you have to change your inclinations towards food. It should be viewed as fuel for the body, yet not as an obsession. To have a productive weight loss, you have to have a way of life change, choosing the right sustenance choices and remaining with those choices for the length of your life.

Tip 5

Weight loss isn't just about numbers. When dieting, don't fear the scales. As the scale's numbers go down, fulfillment goes up. Regardless, when the numbers don't switch or go up, it ends up being anything yet challenging to give up and surrender. Know this; if your weight isn't changing as you need, your body is; the heart improves your mind and cuts down your cholesterol levels. You'll get increasingly thin, and your articles of clothing will start to fit much better. When you begin to find joy in these barely noticeable subtleties, you need to keep getting more slender!

CHAPTER THIRTEEN: 318 POSITIVE AFFIRMATIONS FOR WEIGHT LOSS

Weight loss affirmations can be extraordinarily integral assets to assist you in improving your wellbeing and trim your body. Be that as it may, similarly as significant — they help you to love and acknowledge your body as it as of now seems to be.

Pick around five weight loss and five certainty affirmations from the rundown underneath and state for all to hear every one of them for the entire 5 minutes during the day. That would be an exercise of 50 minutes each day.

Continue rehashing those ten affirmations for seven days, and afterward move onto new ones. Put genuine force and feelings in your voice and remain PERSISTENT!

If you continue doing this, and if you join it with some customary exercises and healthy food, I ensure that you will accomplish the ideal body weight and shape! There's no other way!

We should make a plunge...

Rundown of 318 Positive Affirmations for Weight Loss

1.   I have faith in my capacity to love and acknowledge myself for who I am.

2.   I set myself liberated from all the blame I haul around the food I picked before.

3.   Every day I am practicing and dealing with my body.

4.   Healing is occurring in both my body and mind.

5.   Every time I breathe in, new vitality fills my general existence, and each time I breathe out, all poisons and body fat leave my body.

6.   My wellbeing is improving increasingly more consistently, as is my body.

7.   Everything I eat recuperates and feeds my body, which causes me to arrive at the ideal weight.

8.   I am closer and closer to my ideal weight every single day.

9.   I am so glad and thankful since I weigh _____ kilograms/pounds. (Fill in the ideal number)

10. I can do this; I am doing this; my body is losing weight right at this point.

11. I am relinquishing any blame I hold around food.

12. Eating healthy foods enables my body to get the entirety of the supplements; it should be fit as a fiddle.

13. I am closer and closer to my ideal weight every single day.

14. I feel my craving for fat-rich foods dissolving.

15. I have a compelling impulse to eat just healthy foods, and let go of any prepared foods.

16. I am simply the best form, and I am working hard to turn out to be far and away superior. I will lose weight because I need to, and I have the ability to do this.

17. My body is my sanctuary, and I mindfully deal with it consistently by eating just healthy foods that mend and sustain me.

18. I am mindful that my digestion is working in my preferred position by helping me in putting on my ideal weight.

19. I am accomplishing and keeping up my ideal weight.

20. I have the ability to handily control my weight through a mix of healthy eating and working out.

21.   I am thankful of my body for all the things it accomplishes for me.

22.   Every cell in my body is healthy and fit, as am I.

23.   I feel my body losing weight in every snapshot of the day.

24.   I always bite my food appropriately with the goal that my body can process it and take out the supplements I have to lose weight.

25.   I have faith in my capacity to change my habits and make new, positive ones.

26.   I no longer want to stuff my body with unhealthy foods, and I can undoubtedly oppose allurements.

27.   I appreciate life by remaining fit and keeping up my ideal weight.

28.   I am equipped to accomplish my weight loss goals, and I won't let anything remain in my way up to that point.

29.   I acknowledge my body precisely the way it is, and I continually work on improving it.

30.   I totally comprehend that unhealthy foods don't assist me with losing weight, so I eat just healthy nutritious foods.

31.   My digestion rate is at its ideal level, and this

encourages me to arrive at my ideal body weight.

32. I love and favor myself.

33. I am content with my body, heart, and soul.

34. Every day, I am feeling more beneficial and more grounded.

35. I am figuring out how to love my body.

36. It's safe for me to act naturally.

37. Today, I center around the good things that are unfurling in my life.

38. Trusting my body is getting simpler and simpler.

39. Healing is going on in my body and my mind.

40. I decide to breathe in relaxation and breathe out the pressure.

41. My wellbeing is improving, as is my life.

42. I am encircled and secured by the recuperating white light.

43. Everything I eat mends me and feeds me.

44. Making small changes is getting simpler for me.

45. Healing occurs with each child step I take.

46. I am picking progress over flawlessness.

47. My instinct guides me. I realize what to eat and how to carry on with my life.

48. I usually associate with other similar, positive people.

49. Letting go of the past is right for me. It is OK for me to give up.

50. I can feel that everything is starting to change.

51. I am feeling healthy, engaged, and decided.

52. Lots of new and energizing things are opening up in my life.

53. I can recuperate my body. I am recovering my body. My body is mending.

54. I can do this. I am doing this. Mending is going on right at this point.

55. I am guided by a higher force.

56. I am vivacious and solid.

57. I see the best in everybody and then in me.

58. I have faith in my capacity to genuinely love myself for who I am.

59. I acknowledge my body shape and recognize the magnificence it holds.

60.   I am the maker of my future and the driver of my mind.

61.   I let go of unhelpful examples of conduct around food.

62.   I permit myself to settle on decisions and choices for my higher good.

63.   I let go of any blame I hold around food decisions.

64.   I acknowledge my body for the shape I have been honored with.

65.   I let go of connections that are no longer for my higher good.

66.   I put stock in myself and recognize my enormity.

67.   I permit myself to feel good being me.

68.   I acknowledge myself for who I am.

69.   I bring the characteristics of love into my heart.

70.   I have expectations and sureness about what's to come.

71.   I am thankful of the body I own and everything it accomplishes for me.

72.   I do a good measure of exercise routinely.

73.   My body gets all the supplements it needs.

74. My want for fattening foods is dissolving.

75. I have a compelling impulse to eat just wellbeing giving and nutritious foods.

76. I like myself.

77. I am achieving and keeping up my ideal weight.

78. I am solid and healthy.

79. I am serene and calm.

80. My Mind, Body, and Soul are gifts of the Universe to me.

81. My body is my sanctuary, I love and deals with every day of my life.

82. Every day, inside and out, I am improving myself.

83. I am finding flavorful new foods that make me more advantageous.

84. Achieving my weight-loss objective becomes simpler consistently.

85. I am thankful to have a body fit for working out.

86. I am glad for myself for picking a more advantageous lifestyle.

87. I am encircled by people who empower and bolster me.

88.   After a hard workout, I feel fantastically pleased with my achievement.

89.   I am always centered around liking myself.

90.   Becoming fit gives me a progressively positive point of view.

91.   Every cell in my body feels vigorous and healthy.

92.   I am enchanted that my garments are starting to fit better.

93.   I am finding muscles I didn't realize I had.

94.   I am starting to see another, leaner me in the mirror.

95.   Fitness is turning into energy that I appreciate.

96.   Everywhere I look, I discover others excited for losing weight.

97.   It's anything but difficult to track down fast ways to burn additional calories consistently.

98.   Losing weight causes me to feel progressively sure and OK with myself.

99.   My overabundance fat is softening away to uncover my solid, lean muscles.

100.   The thin internal me is cheerfully developing.

101. I am giving myself the solid, healthy body I merit.

102. Losing weight falls into place without any issues for me.

103. I am joyfully accomplishing my weight loss goals.

104. I am losing weight each day.

105. I love to exercise consistently.

106. I am eating foods that add to my wellbeing and prosperity.

107. I eat just when I am ravenous.

108. I currently obviously observe myself at my ideal weight.

109. I love the flavor of healthy food.

110. I am in charge of the amount I eat.

111. I am getting a charge out of working out; it causes me to feel great.

112. I am turning out to be fitter and more grounded every day through exercise.

113. I am effectively reaching and keeping up my ideal weight

114. I love and care for my body.

115. I have the right to have a thin, healthy, appealing body.

116. I am growing increasingly healthy dietary patterns constantly.

117. I am getting slimmer consistently.

118. I look and feel extraordinary.

119. I take the necessary steps to be healthy.

120. I am joyfully re-imagined achievement.

121. I decide to exercise.

122. I need to eat foods that cause me to look and to feel good.

123. I am answerable for my wellbeing.

124. I love my body.

125. I am quiet with making my better body.

126. I am joyfully practicing each morning when I wake up intending to arrive at the weight loss that I need.

127. I am investing in my weight loss program by changing my dietary patterns from unhealthy to healthy.

128. I am content with each part I do in my extraordinary exertion to lose weight.

129. Every day, I am getting slimmer and more beneficial.

130. I am building up an alluring body.

131. I am building up a lifestyle of lively wellbeing.

132. I am making a body that I like and appreciate.

133. My lifestyle eating changes are changing my body.

134. I am feeling incredible since I have lost more than 10 pounds in about a month and can hardly wait to meet my woman companion.

135. I have a level stomach.

136. I commend my own capacity to make choices around food.

137. I am joyfully gauging 20 pounds less.

138. I like to walk 3 to 4 times per week and do conditioning exercises at any rate 3 times per week.

139. I take 8 glasses of water a day.

140. I eat products of the soil day by day and eat, for the most part, chicken and fish.

141. I am learning and utilizing the psychological, emotional, and profound abilities for progress. I will change!

142.   I will make new thoughts about myself and my body.

143.   I love and value my body.

144.   It's energizing to find my remarkable food and exercise framework for weight loss.

145.   I am a weight loss example of overcoming adversity.

146.   I am charmed to be the ideal weight for me.

147.   It's simple for me to follow a solid food plan.

148.   I decide to grasp thoughts of trust in my capacity to make positive changes in my life.

149.   It feels great to move my body. Exercise is entertaining!

150.   I utilize deep breathing to assist me with relaxing and handle stress.

151.   I am a beautiful individual.

152.   I have the right to be at my ideal weight.

153.   I am an adorable individual. I merit love. It is OK for me to lose weight.

154.   I am a solid nearness on the planet at my lower weight.

155. I discharge the need to condemn my body.

156. I acknowledge and make the most of my sexuality. It's OK to feel exotic.

157. My digestion is incredible.

158. I keep up my body with ideal wellbeing.

159. I totally and completely love and acknowledge myself.

160. I appreciate a solid mind-body association.

161. Every day, I develop more in love with my body.

162. I am thankful of all my body accomplishments for me.

163. I am liberated from the blame of poor dietary habits of the past.

164. My wellbeing improves every single day.

165. I appreciate sustaining solid foods.

166. I am constantly shriveling every day.

167. Healing is happening in my mind, body, and soul.

168. I discharge any blame I hold around food.

169. I feel staggeringly hot at my normal weight of _____ pounds.

170. My body is my haven.

171. I feel my fat cells contracting constantly.

172. I can feel my body sliding into my size ____ pants.

173. I am completely in control of my craving.

174. I am in all-out control of my food choices.

175. Every cell in my body is dynamic and solid.

176. I have the full ability to make solid habits.

177. I appreciate eating gradually to encounter my meals.

178. My want for undesirable foods is lessening every day.

179. I discharge abundance weight from my body.

180. I am the ideal weight for my stature.

181. Keeping fit brings such a great amount of delight into my life.

182. I have a great time exhausting vitality through development.

183. I am fit for arriving at my weight loss goals.

184. My digestion is expedient and productive.

185. I love the sustenance of high vibration foods.

186. My stomach related framework streams easily.

187. I discharge compulsion to eat to overabundance.

188. I love what I see when I look in the mirror.

189. My bends make me so novel.

190. I dress in a way that highlights my highlights.

191. I am positive about my appearance.

192. My dream body is the body I inhabit.

193. I love improving my physical wellness.

194. I am so beautiful.

195. I think that it's simple to lose weight.

196. I appreciate working out.

197. I am naturally thin.

198. I have faith in my capacity to lose weight and keep it off.

199. I have the right to be thin, sound, and glad.

200. I have a natural sound mind and body.

201. I will think positively and just naturally lose weight.

202. I think that it's simple to remain fit as a fiddle.

203.   I love eating well food and supporting my body.

204.   I eat well and set a genuine model for my family.

205.   I value my determination and my capacity to deal with my weight.

206.   I've set up a normal exercise conspire that I can follow without any problem.

207.   I'm grateful for the people who assist me with accomplishing my definitive goals of weight loss.

208.   I can, without much of a stretch, occupy myself from eateries and offices that can be utilized as a compulsion to rehearse undesirable eating habits.

209.   I have built up another good dieting habit.

210.   I decide to be attractive and fit.

211.   My mind is hard-wired to need just solid food, and my body feels that physical activity is important day by day.

212.   Every day I eat well nutritious food.

213.   With each progression I take, mending occurs.

214.   My body exploits the sound food I eat.

215.   My dream life is drawing nearer and closer to me consistently; I'm alive.

216.   All inversions on my way to significance are just transitory.

217.   Everything is feasible for me.

218.   I can make supernatural occurrences all the time.

219.   I can and will achieve all of my goals, be they well off, great, or glad.

220.   Even the littlest move is the start of an epic excursion, and even the littlest advancement towards my goals is justified, despite all the trouble.

221.   On this Earth, no test is unreasonably difficult for me to survive.

222.   I invite everyday difficulties because I realize that is the thing that makes me more grounded.

223.   I am not my past, and my past isn't me.

224.   I'm encompassed by people who need me to accomplish my goals.

225.   To me, every single obstruction is a learning experience.

226.   My way to joy is simple because I recognize what I truly need and incentive in life.

227.   I head to sleep around evening time, understanding that I put my best exertion today.

228.   The Law of Attraction affirmation is my ally, and I can polarize anything I need, and I decide to charge wellbeing and health in my life.

229.   I decide to exercise.

230.   Exercising feels great.

231.   The more that I move, the more grounded that I feel.

232.   It is simple for me to follow a good dieting plan.

233.   I have control over how much food I eat.

234.   Every day I get more grounded and slimmer.

235.   I'm glad to accomplish my goals and get slimmer consistently.

236.   I am burning calories consistently.

237.   Healing happens in my body, just as in my mind.

238.   I am burning calories every single day.

239.   I am an adorable individual.

240.   I simply eat what I need.

241.   I have the right to be thin, sound, and to feel appealing.

242.   I'm eating food for my new weight.

243. I'm constantly creating more beneficial eating habits.

244. I treat my body with consideration and love.

245. I merit my ideal weight.

246. Getting solid is my aspiration, and I can achieve it.

247. Changes in my lifestyle change my body.

248. I acknowledge my body.

249. I utilize my psychological and emotional capacities to get achievement.

250. I have confidence and trust later on.

251. I am the maker of my future and the driver of my mind

252. I just permit positive thoughts in my mind.

253. I'm glad, and I'm encircled by acceptable people.

254. I can change my life.

255. I'm arranged to make new thoughts regarding myself and my body.

256. I am focused on my goals.

257. I can make positive changes in my life.

258.   I believe in myself and my capacity to succeed.

259.   I can lose weight.

260.   I will lose weight.

261.   I can do anything I need in life.

262.   I decide to be solid.

263.   I put stock in myself.

264.   I grasp smart dieting and exercise.

265.   I can do this, and I am doing it.

266.   I'm thin, sound and solid.

267.   I eat what I need, when I need and stop when I begin to feel full.

268.   I am feeding my body with new foods and water.

269.   I make the most of my food and eat mindfully.

270.   I appreciate discovering more ways to get increasingly dynamic.

271.   I love moving my body and getting dynamic at this point.

272.   I tune in to what my body needs with love.

273.   I love and acknowledge myself now.

274. Every day I draw nearer to my ideal weight.

275. I eat everything mindfully and gradually, and I appreciate each nibble.

276. I'm now the sort of individual who can accomplish my ideal weight and solid living goals without much of a stretch.

277. I make conscious decisions that assist me with accomplishing my ideal weight.

278. I'm improving my wellbeing consistently.

279. Every day I get slimmer, more beneficial and fitter.

280. I love my body.

281. I love and regard my body now and always.

282. Being sound and thin is simple for me now.

283. Being sound and thin is a top need for me now.

284. Every day I make solid choices for myself.

285. Being solid and thin gets simpler for me consistently.

286. I love and support my body and mind.

287. I'm equipped for accomplishing my ideal weight, and consistently it gets simpler and simpler.

288.   I'm solid and upbeat.

289.   I truly appreciate moving my body now.

290.   I love and value all aspects of my body now.

291.   I'm appreciating incorporating extremely sound habits with my life.

292.   I love drinking water and strolling.

293.   I make sure that I exercise every day.

294.   I work on my mindset to assist me with feeling extremely positive.

295.   I have the stuff to accomplish my ideal weight.

296.   I love and regard my body now.

297.   I eat mindfully now.

298.   I am my ideal weight, shape, and size.

299.   I am looking and feeling my best.

300.   I love myself precisely as I am.

301.   Every day and inside and out, my habits bolster the best form of me.

302.   I am thankful for what I look like and how I feel.

303.   I effectively and easily accomplish and keep up my ideal weight, shape, and size.

304.   I eat anything I desire. I naturally prefer foods that are exceptionally nutritious and low carb/low calorie or.

305.   I eat what I need, and I prefer (x, y, and z type foods).

306.   The first taste is always the best; after that (food type) goes downhill.

307.   Nothing tastes on a par with meager feels.

308.   I am fit, solid, and awesome.

309.   I love solid, healthy foods that are beneficial for me inside and out.

310.   I am easily making positive, solid choices for my life and my body.

311.   I love to move, exercise, and remain fit as a fiddle.

312.   Exercise makes me feel solid, imperative, and alive.

313.   I react to an emotional miracle in sound ways.

314.   Food is fuel. My body is the sanctuary that houses my soul. I treat it with care and regard energizing myself with foods that are spotless, nutritious, and healthy.

315.   I search for ways to be dynamic, fit, and sound.

316.   I am effectively keeping up my weight of _____

and size _____.

317.   My garments look and feel great on me.

318.   Beauty emanates from within me. What I look like is simply good to beat all.

Some Final Words

Activity is the way to progress. Simply the perusing won't benefit you in any way. So pay attention to this! Begin utilizing affirmations consistently in your life and don't disregard the standard physical exercises and even diet. Great outcomes are inescapable. Yet, if you choose to stop and simply do what you've been doing as long as you can remember, there's no way around it.

Just we are liable for our outcomes and for the outcomes we get. You can currently pick "where to" from here. I trust you'll make an intelligent choice.

CHAPTER FOURTEEN: WEIGHT LOSS CHANGING HABITS

Weight control is tied in with rolling out little improvements that you can live with forever. As you fuse these minor changes into your lifestyle, you'll start to perceive how they can indicate big calorie savings and weight loss. Here are my best ten habits to assist you with transforming your fantasy of weight loss into a reality:

1. Assess your eating habits

Is it accurate to say that you are eating late around evening time, snacking while at the same time cooking, completing the children's meals? Investigate, and it will be anything but difficult to identify a couple of practices you can change that will mean big calorie savings.

2. If you neglect to plan, plan to come up short

You need a methodology for your meals and tidbits. Pack invigorating snacks for the times of day that you realize you are normally ravenous and can, without much of a stretch, wanderer from your eating plan.

3. Always shop with a full tummy

It's a catastrophe waiting to happen to go into the market when you are eager. Shop from a readied list, so drive purchasing is kept to a base. Eating right beginnings with loading sound food in your washroom and cooler.

4. Eat customary meals

Make sense of the recurrence of your meals that work best in your life and stick to it. Standard meals help prevent gorging.

5. Eat your food taking a seat at a table and from a plate

Food eaten out of bundles and keeping in mind that standing is forgettable. You can end up eating parts more than if you plunk down and consciously make the most of your meals.

6. Serve food onto singular plates, and leave the additional items back at the oven

Bowls of food on the table ask to be eaten, and it takes mind-blowing won't delve in for quite a long time. Keep in mind; it takes around 20 minutes for your mind to get the sign from your gut that you are full.

7. Eat gradually, bite each nibble, and appreciate the flavor of the food

Take a stab at resting your fork among chomps and drinking a lot of water with your meals.

8. Try not to have after supper

This is the place heaps of people pack on the additional pounds. If you are ravenous, have a go at fulfilling your desire with a non-caloric refreshment or a bit of hard sweets. Brushing your teeth after supper helps diminish the compulsion to eat again.

9. If you nibble during the day, treat the bite like a smaller than normal meal

The most nutritious bites contain complex sugars and a limited quantity of protein and fat.

10. Start your day with breakfast. It is the most important meal of the day

In the wake of a monotonous night's rest, your body needs the fuel to get your digestion moving and give you vitality for the remainder of the day.

CHAPTER FIFTEEN: HOW TO USE HYPNOSIS TO CHANGE EATING HABITS

Step by step instructions to Recognize Your Food Addiction

Before you experience the subtleties encompassing hypnosis for overeating, we should discuss food addiction. Disordered eating is the point at which you've built up an undesirable relationship with food and eating.

Here are a couple of signs to pay special mind to that can assist you in deciding whether you have a food addiction.

Weight and Never-ending Worry

We've all felt pressure—by the media just, as by our friends—to look a specific way. Be that as it may, holding yourself up to unreasonable measures of excellence can affect your wellbeing. You may feel forced to diet, which can prompt stressing and binge eating.

You may likewise feel constantly stressed over dieting,

food, and working out.

If you feel blameworthy or embarrassed about the amount you're eating, it can add unnecessary strain to your life.

From Dieting to Disordered Eating

At the point when people feel forced by the media to look a specific way, they begin dieting.

Nonetheless, dieting can leave you engrossed with food. Therefore, you can create disordered eating habits or a food issue. This will set you on a constant dieting/binge eating cycle.

The Constant Cycle

As you become engrossed with food and weight loss, you'll likely build up an undesirable eating design. This example can leave you limiting yourself, skipping meals, binge eating, and afterward dieting once more.

As you yo-yo diet, you'll notice constant changes in your weight.

In time, you may feel like you are stuck in this constant cycle.

The Symptoms

While there are a couple of different eating issue, the general side effects include:

- Eating too rapidly

- Continuing to eat even though you're full

- Hiding food or eating covertly out of blame

- Feeling constrained to eat

- Feeling blameworthy in the wake of overeating

- Eating when you're not eager

Look out for these indications. If you trust you have a food addiction, hypnotherapy for overeating habits can help.

Hypnosis for Overeating: How It Helps

So does hypnosis for overeating truly work?

Indeed! As indicated by this examination, patients getting hypnotherapy for overeating demonstrated more prominent improvement than in any event, 70% of customers accepting nonhypnotic treatment.

Hypnotherapy can assist you in beating your food addiction. Here are a couple of ways hypnotherapy helps to prevent us from overeating.

Mindful Eating

Food addictions cause people to indulge without speculation. It turns into an impulse until we neglect to consider our activities thoroughly.

Hypnosis can show the mind to stay mindful.

You'll figure out how to perceive your desires, how full you feel, and how to stay mindful when you're eating. Mindfulness will keep you mindful of your activities, so you can gain control over when you're eating, the amount you're eating, and how often you eat.

Getting out from under the Habit

After some time, we create formal reasoning. Binge eating makes us address ourselves with negative, destructive thoughts. Accordingly, we end up binge eating again, which causes a constant cycle of binge eating.

Our yearnings, overeating, and stress can trigger these negative thoughts.

During these minutes, calmly inhale and remind yourself all is well. Something else, your stress will transform into nervousness and energize your binge eating.

You need to break these negative thought spirals to end your food addiction.

Hypnosis for overeating can assist you with getting out from under the habit.

Utilizing hypnosis, you can assume responsibility for your thoughts. Rather than suffocating in the negatives, you'll figure out how to transform your subconscious into a partner (not a foe).

Treat the Underlying Condition

Sometimes, food addiction is brought about by another condition.

For instance, you may experience the ill effects of despondency or a tension issue. Such conditions may cause your negative thoughts, which this way energizes your binge eating.

Hypnosis can enable you and give the psychological quality you need to battle these conditions. Rather than permitting your downturn or uneasiness to control your thoughts, you can take control and change the content.

Treating the underlying condition can assist you in stopping your binge eating habits.

Reestablish Your Confidence

An absence of self-certainty can make us freeze up. Rather than making a move or dealing with our negative thoughts, we feel like everything is outside our ability to control.

At the point when we need trust in ourselves, our

negative thoughts can dominate.

Hypnotherapy can assist you with reinforcing your self-certainty. By figuring out how to put stock in yourself, you can reclaim control. That way, you can stop your unfortunate binge eating habits.

With hypnotherapy for overeating, you'll have the self-certainty to defeat anything.

Self-Hypnosis Techniques

Before you begin utilizing hypnotherapy for overeating, you should realize you have a couple of alternatives accessible. For instance, you can think about one-on-one sessions with a trance inducer. You may likewise choose to tune in to hypnotherapy chronicles.

There's additionally self-hypnosis. Here are a couple of methods to assist you get started:

• Note your wellbeing, surveying how you feel toward the start and end of every session

• Breathe deeply to tell your mind and body it's time to relax

• Count down from 10, which tells your mind you're entering a condition of hypnosis

• Speak to yourself utilizing affirmations, or positive recommendations, for example, "I'm liberated from overeating."

• Visualize yourself taking control and carrying on with a more joyful, more beneficial life

With these strategies, you can relax and reframe your mind. Utilizing hypnosis for overeating will help you regain control of your eating habits and by and large life.

Hypnosis for Overeating: Take a Bite of a Healthier Life

Slowly inhale and recollect that you're in control. With hypnosis for overeating, you can find a more advantageous life without disrupting the general flow without your food addiction.

CHAPTER SIXTEEN: A FUNDAMENTAL SELF-HYPNOSIS SESSION FOR WEIGHT LOSS

Because of the considerable number of advantages that self-hypnosis brings to the table, you are going to need to make sense of what your goal is before you start self-hypnosis. For example, you could be doing it just to relax, or you may be attempting to change your way of thinking. A decent way to prepare to accomplish your goal with self-hypnosis is to work out certain affirmations in advance that you can go over in your mind as you enter a condition of a daze. For example:

• "I will put forth a valiant effort on my test tomorrow. I am shrewd, and I will hold all the data that is introduced to me."

• "I am completely fit for accomplishing whatever it might be that I set my focus on. I am in control of my own predetermination, and I am significant and loved."

Stage 1: Prepare Yourself for Hypnosis

Get into something agreeable: When you need to relax at home, you, for the most part, don't attempt to relax in close pants, a secured shirt, or any prohibitive apparel. At the point when you set yourself up for self-hypnosis, you should get into agreeable garments that won't divert you. Focus on the temperature of where you are, as you may need something, for example, a sweater to keep you warm or shorts to keep you cool.

Discover someplace calm: Depending on where you need to situate yourself, you will need to locate a peaceful space. You might need to sit or rest during hypnosis, so locate a decent, agreeable bed, sofa, or seat so you can accomplish mental harmony.

Set aside interruptions: Self-hypnosis has to do with a ton of core interest. Set aside this effort to kill your telephone or any hardware that you have. Entering a dazed period won't be effective if you are around a PC or tuning in to alarms from your telephone.

Stage 2: Enter Hypnosis

Close your eyes: As you close your eyes, attempt to dispose of any stress, dread, or uneasiness that you feel is overloading you. From the outset, you may locate this difficult, yet work to drive those thoughts away. Envision them lifting up from you and coasting away into the air. If you experience difficulty doing this with your eyes closed, you can, on the other hand, pick a point of convergence in your space to concentrate on and permit your eyes to get overwhelming and relaxed.

Relax: There might be a great deal of pressure in your body that you are unconscious of. Start with the base of your feet and work your way up with every one of your body parts gradually discharging pressure. Envision the strain gradually leaking up through your body and evaporating. Picture your body getting lighter with every second. You may think that it's simpler to utilize symbolism procedures, for example, envisioning water surging around your feet or having your body be lifted up from the beginning.

Inhale: Breathing is a significant piece of self-hypnosis. Make sure that you take moderate and deep breaths to discharge any antagonism or strain that might encompass you. Intend to breathe and fill in your lungs with life, vitality, and liveliness.

Envision: Visualizing situations can assist you with accomplishing certain outcomes that you need. For example, if you are hoping to lose weight, consider envisioning yourself shedding pounds by swimming off the weight. You can get as point by point as could be expected under the circumstances; however, make sure you utilize your five detects. You can do this by asking yourself these inquiries: what do I smell, taste, and feel?

Acknowledge: At this point, you should feel relaxed. Set aside this effort to value your condition of relaxation. Envision yourself at the highest point of steps that lead to water. Envision yourself, sliding the steps and developing your body in the tidiness and virtue of the water.

Free yourself: As you plunge into the water, permit yourself to imagine your feet coasting up and your body drifting openly in the water. Describe in your mind what you are doing, and talk in a future tense. Rehash positive explanations, and maintain a strategic distance from any cynicism.

Exit: After you feel relaxed settled, you can consider leaving your condition of hypnosis. Stroll up the steps in your mind from which you have plunged, and keep repeating your positive articulations as you rise up out of the water.

Stage 3: Manifest Your Experience

Now that you have performed self-hypnosis, you will need to invest your amounts of energy into play. There are a lot of ways that you can upgrade your experience to accomplish the express that you sought after.

Mean what you state: For any of the mantras that you expressed during your hypnosis, be certain that you implied them. Put stock in yourself and your activities, because this will assist you with accomplishing your representations.

Physically upgrade your experience: There are certain exercises that you can do while you are in your self-mesmerizing state. Have a go at entwining your fingers together, squirming your toes, or imagine your arms getting substantial.

Utilize external help: Real-world upgrades can likewise be utilized to assist you with accomplishing and enter hypnosis. For example, you can attempt music, timers, or the sound of water or the downpour backwoods to comfort you.

Develop with inspiration: We all have goals in life that we want to accomplish. You can utilize self-hypnosis to enable you to imagine what you might want your life to resemble, and any goals that you may have for yourself. Try not to be reluctant to utilize sleep-inducing procedures to assist you with turning into the individual that you wish to be.

Self-hypnosis is valuable for boosting your certainty, empowering yourself towards a more advantageous lifestyle, and improving your exhibition. Follow these essential strides of self-hypnosis to assist you with moving towards your ideal goals:

Consider what you need to accomplish or change and express your goal in a solitary sentence.

Pick a spot where you can be totally agreeable if you sit in a seat or resting.

Set a time limit by intellectually giving yourself the accompanying proposal: 'Precisely ten minutes from now, my eyelids open naturally and I feel quiet, refreshed and revived.'

Close your eyes and take a couple of deep breaths. Dynamically relax every one of your muscles, from head to toe, or toe to head, whichever you prefer.

Tally down from ten to one and disclose to yourself that with each number, you'll turn out to be progressively relaxed, both physically and intellectually, and go deeper into a stupor.

At the point when you're in a deepened stupor state, begin utilizing the goal explanation you contrived for your self-hypnosis session. Recollect your single sentence goal proclamation, and make it as distinctive as conceivable in your creative mind. At that point, let go. Trust that you have given it over to your unconscious mind and that this clever piece of you will presently take care of the issue.

Check yourself alert, up from one to ten, and disclose to yourself that you're no longer in a daze.

A couple of moments in the wake of enlivening from self-hypnosis, you are still in an exceptionally suggestible state. Utilize that time to strengthen how relaxed and quiet you feel, and how satisfied you are that your unconscious mind is helping you reach your goal.

CHAPTER SEVENTEEN: WEIGHT LOSS HYPNOSIS 30 MINUTE AFFIRMATIONS

Not many people have a simple, direct relationship with food. For the majority of us, food conveys meaning. We partner certain foods with holidays and festivities—and the other way around.

A considerable lot of us additionally eat as a way to calm emotional distress. After a baffling, defeating, or stressful day, a considerable lot of us go after "comfort food"— unhealthy, high-fat tidbits and treats that just bring temporary help. Sometimes, we realize we are eating emotionally. Different times, we eat mindlessly, uninformed of what is driving our longings and impulses.

Hypnosis for weight loss hinders emotional eating by upsetting the connections between specific feelings and foods. As you enter a relaxed stupor state, you will turn out to be distinctly mindful of your thoughts, encompassing weight, exercise, and food. You can understand that they are only that—thoughts. Only thoughts with no natural worth or truth. At that point, you can take advantage of your inward intelligence, find that you do have choices, and use your capacity to build up new thoughts and convictions.

How about we take a gander at a quick guide to perceive how the procedure may search for you?

Your unconscious mind may believe that you can't handle stress, and treats can relieve stress. Hypnosis permits you to identify, challenge, and supplant that conviction. You can handle stress. Treats don't relieve stress (and may even trigger feelings of disgrace and blame, bringing about stress, yet additionally feelings of misery and annihilation). Furthermore, other positive activities, such as reflection, workmanship, or exercise, can relieve stress all the more effectively and improve your emotional well-being over the long haul.

Through hypnosis, you can reframe the narratives you are letting yourself know and change your relationship with feelings, yearning, and food. You can find what you, as an individual, need to sustain your physical body and inward world.

"I do realize that I presently have control over food. I eat when I'm ravenous, and, more often than not, I stop when I'm full. Without a doubt, I have a cheat to a great extent; however, it's quite often a conscious choice, and it doesn't crash my whole diet. It doesn't even wreck my day. I'm ready to get directly back on target — something I'd never had the option to do."

By speaking with your subconscious mind, you can

make conscious decisions about your diet and exercise schedule. What's more, even more profoundly, you can isolate food from feelings and cut off the connection between what you eat and your feeling of self-worth.

Basic Questions About Weight Loss Hypnosis

Does Hypnosis Reduce or Eliminate Cravings?

Yearnings are ordinary and nothing to be embarrassed about. In any case, longings can turn into an issue when they begin to coordinate your decisions.

Hypnosis decreases their force and impact, denying impulses of their capacity instead of wiping out desires. When craving for a treat emerges, you will have the option to delay, reflect, and choose if that treat truly serves your drawn-out needs.

It's tied in with perceiving that while we feel like accomplishing something, we don't need to act that out."

Will It Make Me Hate Foods I Love?

No. Hypnosis isn't tied in with removing delights and joys! It's tied in with helping you relish them consciously and with some restraint. Although you love a specific food, you may not love how you feel after eating a lot of it (or eating it time and again).

The best hypnosis depends on positive saying: "For my body, a lot of food is harming. I need my body to live. I owe my body regard and security."

Hypnosis welcomes you to reframe your reasoning and genuinely, deeply accept that your body—and your entire self—merits joy and well-being.

Does It Just Make Me Want to Eat Healthier?

Hypnosis does considerably more than just launch a craving for more beneficial eating. It will likewise assist you with building self-regard and certainty, permitting you to confide in yourself and finish on your goals.

Hypnosis doesn't simply address issues on a superficial level. It works deeply, mending old injuries and creating new ways to health and self-strengthening.

Will I Be Programmed to Eat a Certain Diet?

Hypnosis is anything but a one-size-fits-all diet plan—or a diet plan by any stretch of the imagination!— and you won't be programmed to eat a specific way. Rather, you will become familiar with your interesting dietary needs and how to adjust your unconscious mind to what your conscious mind definitely thinks about sustenance.

Most significantly, you will guarantee another feeling of office over your eating with the goal that your food choices are conscious, not mindless, or emotionally determined.

Do I Need to Exercise in Addition to Eating Better?

Exercise is quite often an awesome expansion to any lifestyle change or self-care schedule. While you can surely lose weight through diet alone, working out can assist you with interfacing with your body and lift your state of mind.

Notwithstanding burning calories, exercise adds to heart well-being, muscle tone, and general physical, mental, and emotional well-being.

To what extent Does Weight Loss Hypnosis Take?

To what extent before I can get started? You can begin hypnosis for weight loss when you like!

If you are worried that another emotional wellness issue or conclusion could meddle with your weight loss or hypnosis process, connect with your PCP and essential specialist first. While you might be anxious to begin, it's imperative to make sure that hypnosis is a protected, effective decision for you.

You can likewise look for hypnosis sessions that are specially outfitted to uneasiness, wretchedness, sleep deprivation, and different issues that might be hindering your way to weight loss.

Keep in mind, enduring change originates from recuperating from the back to front.

To what extent Does an Individual Session Take?

Hypnosis chronicles usually take around 20–30 minutes. A live session with an advisor will most likely take about 60 minutes.

Because you will be in a stupor state for most, if not all, of every session, you're probably going to find that the time appears to fly by.

To what extent Before I Start Noticing Results?

The individuals who are especially open to hypnosis will probably start seeing changes to their mindsets in as meager as one session. For a great many people, it takes one to three sessions to see inward enhancements.

You will probably start to see physical changes as your mindset changes. After the main seven day stretch of battling desires and eating mindfully, you may see improvement on the scale.

Be that as it may, hypnosis doesn't accelerate weight loss—it is anything but a convenient solution or crash diet. Hypnosis enables you to make sound, durable changes. If you stay with it and coordinate new eating and exercise habits, you can see genuine physical changes within a month.

Furthermore, not at all like weight loss in a trend diet, these pounds won't creep back on.

To what extent Should I Stick With It?

Your advisor will probably urge you to go to six sessions if you choose face-to-face hypnotherapy.

If you prefer hypnosis chronicles, you should listen every day, in any event, seven days.

Numerous people who have utilized hypnosis for weight loss keep going to sessions or tuning in to accounts, even in the wake of arriving at their underlying goals. This can fill in as a boost, inside registration, and way to alleviation during an especially stressful or difficult day.

All through the procedure, make sure to be patient and kind with yourself. You have the right to give your mind and body the time they need to shift, recuperate, and change.

Utilizing Weight Loss Affirmations

The Power Of Autohypnosis

To accomplish your ideal weight utilizing weight loss affirmations is something other than conceivable. By using weight loss affirmations, you're creating a psychological pathway along which your conscious mind transmits it acutely felt want to lose weight into your subconscious, which holds within it the ability to change or improve any part of your life.

We could state that these encouraging statements resemble portions of software you download every day into the boundlessly ground-breaking PC that is your subconscious, the goal being to reconstruct the subconscious so that it will at the appointed time wipe out from your mindset any negative thoughts or feelings you have which cause you to gorge.

Repeating an everyday affirmation really takes after a gentle type of indoctrinating procedure. Government officials and enormous organizations use TV and other media to rehash their "mantras," specific key expressions - affirmations - which they use to advance their message or brand.

As an individual, you can utilize weight loss affirmations and self-hypnosis in a substantially more effective and direct way to understand your goal. In this case, your cerebrum, or all the more precisely your subconsciousness, is being "washed" by you and your special affirmations that come from your one of a kind conscious of losing weight.

Weight Loss Affirmations

Self-hypnosis may be best under conditions of protection, calm, and relaxation. After you've picked which one of the incredible affirmations recorded beneath is best for you, put aside 15-30 minutes consistently or evening - for half a month - to be distant from everyone else and get relaxed.

Rests, preferably on a bed, and let your arms, hands, and legs become limp. Begin to inhale routinely and decently profoundly, at that point, focus on some point simply over your typical scope of vision; at that point, gradually let them close. Proceed with breathing reasonably and deeply, let your muscles start to extricate from your feet up to your neck, and, afterward, fill your mind with some pictures you partner with relaxation and serenity while breathing gradually and allowing your muscles to muscles.

Mental Imagery

At this point - following 5-10 minutes - you ought to be deeply relaxed and now a lot "closer" to your subconscious and everything that it can accomplish for you.

Presently think about a picture of yourself as you need to be thin, fit, and solid, and afterward, keep up that picture of yourself in your mind.

When your mind is loaded up with this picture of yourself as you need to be, at that point, start to state or murmur to yourself your picked affirmation. Rehash the affirmation, gradually and purposely, around 20 - 30 times - though you don't need to tally - at the same time, keeping up the picture of yourself as thin, solid, and sound in your mind. Sooner or later - you'll naturally know when - you can stop utilizing the affirmation and continuously take yourself back to ordinary consciousness.

If you follow this methodology, precisely, determinedly, and consistently for half a month, you'll before long, find that your hunger has recognizably reduced and that you're losing enthusiasm for sweet and low-quality nourishment. That, joined with a typical degree of physical movement, will bring about significant weight loss and a huge lift to your mental and emotional prosperity.

Be that as it may, utilizing weight loss affirmations along these lines could be depicted as self-hypnosis in the most difficult way possible. By tuning in to a hypnosis download from your pc or mp3 player, you get rid of the need to keep up an adequate degree of consciousness to keep up the verbal reiteration of the affirmation. With a download or mp3, the recommendations are originating from outside and are simpler to absorb and give sink access to your subconscious, and that, joined with your day by day deep relaxation and representation, will, in general, produce results all the more rapidly.

In any case, if you need to utilize the two strategies, here is a rundown of weight loss related affirmations:

- I'm thin and solid and appealing.

- I'm solid, sound, and thin.
- I'm fit, sound, and brimming with vitality.
- I am thin, sound, and pleased with my body.
- I'm thin, beautiful, and sound.
- I'm sound, light, and brimming with vitality.

Expressions of Power

It will be ideal if you note that the entirety of the weight loss affirmations contained in the above rundown of affirmations refer to a circumstance where you're envisioning and avowing, so that recommends that you have what you need. Use weight loss affirmations so that you feel and genuinely envision yourself as being as thin as you need to be. The subconscious doesn't differentiate between what is as of now genuine and what is being pictured, and thus will act promptly to begin making the truth that is being imagined.

CHAPTER EIGHTEEN: RAPID WEIGHT LOSS, FAST BURN AND CALORIE BLAST WITH SELF-HYPNOSIS AND MEDITATION

While there are unlimited diets, enhancements, and supper substitution plans professing to guarantee fast weight loss, most come up short on any scientific proof.

These systems incorporate working out, monitoring calorie consumption, intermittent fasting, and decreasing the number of carbohydrates in the diet.

Techniques for weight loss that scientific examination bolsters incorporate the accompanying:

1. Attempting intermittent fasting

A few examination sponsored methodologies can help weight loss, one of which is intermittent fasting (IF).

Intermittent fasting (IF) is an example of eating that includes standard transient fasts and expending dinners within a shorter period during the day.

A few examinations have shown that momentary

intermittent fasting, which is as long as 24 weeks in span, prompts weight loss in overweight people.

The most widely recognized intermittent fasting strategies incorporate the accompanying:

Interchange day fasting: Fast every other day and eat typically on non-fasting days. The modified form includes eating only 25–30 percent of the body's vitality needs on fasting days.

The 5:2 Diet: Fast on 2 out of at regular intervals. On fasting days, eat 500–600 calories.

The 16/8 technique: Fast for 16 hours and eat just during an 8-hour window. For the vast majority, the 8-hour window would associate with an early afternoon to 8 p.m. A study on this strategy found that eating during a limited period brought about the members expending fewer calories and getting thinner.

It is ideal to embrace a good dieting design on non-fasting days and to maintain a strategic distance from over-eating.

2. Following your diet and exercise

If somebody needs to get more fit, they ought to know about everything that they eat and drink every day. The best method to do this is to log each thing that they devour, in either a diary or an online food tracker.

One study found that following physical movement assisted with weight loss. In the interim, an audit study found a positive relationship between weight loss and the recurrence of checking food admission and exercise. Even a gadget basic as a pedometer can be a helpful weight-loss device.

3. Eating carefully

Careful eating is where people focus on how and where they eat food. This training can empower people to appreciate the food they eat and maintain a stable weight.

As many people have occupied existence, they regularly will, in general, eat rapidly on the run, in the vehicle, working in their work areas, and sitting in front of the TV. Subsequently, numerous people are scarcely mindful of the food they are eating.

Procedures for careful eating include:

Plunking down to eat, preferably at a table: Pay thoughtfulness regarding the food and appreciate the experience.

Staying away from interruptions while eating: Do not turn on the TV, or a PC or telephone.

Eating gradually: Take time to bite and enjoy the food. This method helps with weight loss, as it gives an individual's cerebrum sufficient opportunity to perceive the signs that they are full, which can help prevent over-eating.

Settling on thought about food decisions: Choose foods that are brimming with supporting supplements and those that will fulfill for a considerable length of time as opposed to minutes.

4. Having protein for breakfast

Protein can control hunger hormones to assist people with feeling full. This is, for the most part, because of a reduction in the yearning hormone ghrelin and an ascent in the satiety hormones peptide YY, GLP-1, and cholecystokinin.

Examination on youthful grown-ups has additionally shown that the hormonal impacts of having a high-protein breakfast can keep going for a few hours.

Good decisions for a high-protein breakfast incorporate eggs, oats, nut and seed margarine, quinoa porridge, sardines, and chia seed pudding.

5. Decreasing sugar and refined carbohydrates

It can assist with trading high-sugar snacks for products of the soil.

The Western diet is progressively high in included

sugars, and this has distinct connects to heftiness, even when the sugar happens in refreshments as opposed to food.

Refined carbohydrates are intensely prepared foods that no longer contain fiber and different supplements. These incorporate white rice, bread, and pasta.

These foods rush to process, and they convert to glucose quickly.

Overabundance glucose enters the blood and incites the hormone insulin, which advances fat stockpiling in the fatty tissue. This adds to weight gain.

Where possible, people should trade handled and sugary foods for increasingly fortifying choices. Good food trades include:

- entire grain rice, bread, and pasta rather than the white forms
- natural product, nuts, and seeds rather than high-sugar snacks
- herb teas and natural product imbued water rather than high-sugar soft drinks
- smoothies with water or milk rather than natural product juice

6. Eating much fiber

Dietary fiber depicts plant-based carbohydrates that it is beyond the realm of imagination to expect to process in the small digestive tract, in contrast to sugar and starch. Remembering much fiber for the diet can expand the sentiment of totality, conceivably prompting weight loss.

7. Adjusting gut bacteria

One growing region of examination is concentrating on the job of bacteria in the gut on weight management.

The human gut has a tremendous number and assortment of microorganisms, including around 37 trillion bacteria.

Each individual has different assortments and measures of bacteria in their gut. A few kinds can build the measure of vitality that the individual harvests from food, prompting fat affidavit and weight gain.

A few foods can expand the number of good bacteria in the gut, including:

A wide assortment of plants: Increasing the number of natural products, vegetables, and grains in the diet will bring about an expanded fiber take-up and a progressively various arrangement of gut bacteria. People should attempt to guarantee that vegetables and other plant-based foods contain 75 percent of their supper.

Aged foods: These upgrade the capacity of good bacteria while restraining the development of awful bacteria. Sauerkraut, kimchi, kefir, yogurt, tempeh, and miso all contain good measures of probiotics, which help to build good bacteria. Specialists have examined kimchi generally, and study results recommend that it has hostile to weight impacts. Also, contemplates have indicated that kefir may assist with advancing weight loss in overweight ladies.

Prebiotic foods: These invigorate the development and action of a portion of the good bacteria that guide weight control. Prebiotic fiber happens in numerous soil products, particularly chicory root, artichoke, onion, garlic, asparagus, leeks, banana, and avocado. It is likewise in grains, for example, oats and grain.

8. Getting a pleasant evening's sleep

Various investigations have demonstrated that getting under 5–6 hours of sleep for every night is related to an expanded rate of stoutness. There are a few explanations for this.

Exploration proposes that deficient or low quality sleep hinders the procedure wherein the body changes over calories to vitality, called digestion. At the point when digestion is less compelling, the body may store unused vitality as fat. Moreover, poor sleep can expand the creation of insulin and cortisol, which additionally brief fat stockpiling.

To what extent somebody sleeps additionally influences the guideline of the craving controlling hormones leptin and ghrelin. Leptin imparts signs of completion to the mind.

9. Dealing with your feelings of anxiety

Open-air exercises can help with pressure management.

Stress triggers the arrival of hormones, for example, adrenaline and cortisol, which at first lessening the craving as a feature of the body's battle or flight reaction.

Be that as it may, when people are under steady pressure, cortisol can stay in the circulatory system for more, which will build their hunger and possibly lead to them eating more.

Cortisol flags the need to recharge the body's healthful stores from the preferred wellspring of fuel, which is sugar.

Insulin, at that point, ships the sugar from carbohydrates from the blood to the muscles and cerebrum. If the individual doesn't utilize this sugar in battle or flight, the body will store it as fat.

Specialists found that executing an 8-week stress-management mediation program brought about a significant decrease in the body mass file (BMI) of overweight and hefty youngsters and youths.

CHAPTER NINETEEN: LOSING WEIGHT LOSS FAST AND NATURALLY WITH HYPNOSIS

Would you like to lose weight forever?

Do you set the weight back on when you quit dieting?

Okay, prefer to stop the ceaseless cycle of diets?

In this way, let me give you how hypnosis for weight loss truly works.

Hypnosis for weight loss truly works because it is one of the best ways to lose weight forever.

The examination has demonstrated that hypnosis for weight loss can assist you with losing twice as much weight.

Hypnosis helps you lose weight because it handles the mental explanations behind weight gain.

The best news is that hypnosis is 100% common.

There are no craze diets to follow, pills, or diet enhancements to take.

Hypnosis for weight loss truly works because it depends on four simple standards:

- eat three solid meals a day
- possibly eat when you're ravenous
- quit eating when you feel full
- eat mindfully and appreciate each significant piece of food

Hypnosis for weight loss permits you to eat the food you like.

No food is prohibited.

You figure out how to eat with some restraint and have more control over the amount you eat.

This helps you to decrease the number of calories expended and lose weight naturally.

Hypnosis for weight loss is a delicate way to lose weight naturally and create good dieting habits simultaneously.

Another motivation behind why Hypnosis for weight loss truly works is because it battles emotional eating.

HYPNOTHERAPY CAN BE EXTREMELY EFFECTIVE AT COMBATING EMOTIONAL EATING

Hypnotherapy manages the reason for your emotional eating as opposed to the manifestations.

Development has programmed you to ache for high fat and sugary foods when you are stressed.

You discharge more elevated levels of the hormone cortisol when you are stressed and restless.

Cortisol has numerous advantages; however, one of the effects is it builds your craving for salty, greasy, and sugary foods.

Hypnotherapy can be extremely effective in handling stress and tension, which at that point lessens your cortisol levels, and which thus diminishes your craving for high sugar and salty foods.

If your weight-loss diets have been ineffective previously, there is a decent possibility you didn't manage the emotional reason for your undesirable diet.

Another motivation behind why Hypnosis for weight loss truly works is because it handles comfort eating.

HYPNOTHERAPY CAN BE EXTREMELY EFFECTIVE AT

DEALING WITH COMFORT EATING

Eating is one of life's normal delights.

At the point when you eat, your body discharges the 'feel-great' substance serotonin.

It is nothing unexpected that you feel great when you eat.

Be that as it may, this can prompt a vicious cycle of eating to feel great when you feel low.

You are bound to gain weight if you eat to feel great when you feel sad.

Eating to decrease sadness prompts lament and blame because you are not accomplishing your weight loss goals.

This, thus, expands those feelings of misery.

Eating along these lines doesn't assist you with managing the reason for your sadness.

Emotional eating just aggravates your feelings of sadness.

It negatively influences your feelings about your body picture, making you feel sad again.

That is the point at which your self-defeating 'internal voice' kicks in and lets you know there isn't any point adhering to your diet.

You end up caught in a vicious cycle.

Another explanation that shows hypnosis for weight loss truly works is because it improves your self-regard and body picture.

HYPNOTHERAPY CAN HELP WITH YOUR BODY IMAGE AND SELF-ESTEEM

It is expressing the undeniable that your self-picture endures when you gain weight.

Exploration has indicated that hypnotherapy can improve your body picture, self-regard, and self-worth.

It can inspire you to succeed and lose weight.

You don't need to eat to feel great with developed self-regard and self-worth, so you are bound to adhere to your diet.

Hypnotherapy can assist you with assuming responsibility for your hunger.

It can assist you with feeling quiet and give you better vitality levels.

It can assist you with halting utilizing food as a way of dealing with stress, particularly when you are feeling stressed, exhausted, or restless.

If you eat close to nothing or an excessive amount of your well-being, personal satisfaction can be influenced.

This can make you have negative feelings towards food.

Hypnotherapy can help you settle on more beneficial choices and control urgent eating, gorging, and weight gain.

The issue with most thinning diets is they don't manage the mental issues that cause you to gorge.

When you stop the diet, you will set the weight back on.

Hypnotherapy is different.

It can assist you with getting more fit by, in a general sense, shifting your impression of food and diet.

Heftiness and diabetes levels are rising, and millions are spent on well-being training bringing issues to light on proper dieting.

Many are dependent on lousy nourishment.

Food is addictive.

Examination proposes that hypnotherapy can help the arrival of peptides that control feelings of yearning.

In what capacity CAN HYPNOSIS HELP

ME LOSE WEIGHT FOREVER?

Hypnotherapy can change your impression of food and eating habits, which raises your certainty, inspiration, and versatility levels to assist you with succeeding.

There are six key components to Hypnotherapy Weight Loss that assist you with shedding pounds forever:

#1. Build up THE RIGHT ATTITUDE

You need to be spurred, decided, and headed to lose weight.

Hypnotherapy will help you with having a positive demeanor and trusting you can lose weight and carry on with a healthy life.

It will reframe your reasoning and urge you to assume personal liability for your weight, the executives.

Some portion of the program concentrates on those self-defeating thought designs that may have made you surrender previously.

#2. Create HEALTHY EATING Behaviors

When your mentality is in the opportune spot, and you have started up, the program helps you let go of the unfortunate eating habits and receive progressively smart dieting habits so you can lose weight.

The goal is to assist you with assuming back

responsibility for food and increment your inspiration to carry on with a more advantageous life, including expanding exercise where conceivable.

The program helps you identify unfortunate eating examples and discover ways to change your eating practices.

I will assist you with building up an eating plan that adheres to the 80-20 standard.

You will eat strongly 80% of the time and have a touch of what you lavish for staying 20%.

#3. SET SMALL ACHIEVABLE GOALS

Possibly you might want to be a similar size; you were the point at which you were at school.

In any case, that may mean losing five stone.

Try not to set yourself such an enormous goal.

Break the big goal into small goals.

Set yourself smaller progressively practical goals of 5% or 10% and give yourself an any longer timeframe to accomplish it.

It is essential to give yourself some adaptability too.

There will be high points and low points on your weight loss venture.

Significantly, your weight loss program is adaptable, not unbending; else, it won't feel like it fits into your life.

#4. SET SPECIFIC GOALS

Try not to set summed up goals, for example,

"I should eat less food" or "I should exercise more."

Rather set specific momentary goals, for example,

"I will take a sound lunch to work each day as opposed to setting off to a drive-through eatery."

On the other hand, "I will take a 30-minute stroll with my companion on a Monday and Wednesday evening after work every week".

#5. Have BREAKFAST EVERY DAY

Numerous people skip breakfast because they are excessively occupied or not eager.

Breakfast is one of the most important meals of the day.

Eat moderate vitality discharging foods, for example, oats that will prop you up until lunch.

Set your caution 15 minutes sooner.

Make sure you hit the sack 15 minutes sooner with the goal that you don't decrease your total rest time.

#6. EAT FOOD MINDFULLY

Figure out how to take little nibbles of your food.

Bite every significant piece gradually, focusing your thoughts on the surface, sounds, and kinds of food.

Put down your cutlery between every significant piece to assist you with eating all the more gradually.

Ideally, you ought to go through around 20-minutes eating every meal.

To assist you with changing the time you spend eating, set a timer to realize to what extent you have spent eating.

Thus, if you are keen on getting thinner forever, why not try weight loss hypnosis?

Sympathetically NOTE

Singular outcomes can fluctuate. There is no assurance that hypnotherapy will be effective for each situation. For Hypnosis for weight loss to be effective, you need to be available to change and completely dedicated.

CHAPTER TWENTY: THE DANGEROUS SIDE OF HYPNOSIS

Hypnosis is an exceptionally unique device that allows us to take advantage of the human mind's shocking intensity in the quest for positive, dynamic, and lasting change. Hypnosis can be utilized to accomplish anything from simple certainty support for a driving test or other test, through stopping habits like smoking or nail gnawing, and going on to distinct supernatural occurrence fixes like helping somebody become ready to travel alone through the outback of Australia, in the wake of being caught inside with agoraphobia for a considerable length of time. We know beyond what most exactly how effective Hypnosis can be; however, there are restrictions to its capacity. Inconceivabilities remain difficulties, and Hypnosis isn't a supernatural occurrence remedy for anything, despite what a few people may guarantee. So it is critical to get that: Hypnosis can't fix innate harm or hereditary issues. Hypnosis can't prevent the maturing procedure or make you live forever. Hypnosis can't assist you with accomplishing whatever is really physically unthinkable. Sometimes Hypnosis can seem to do incredible things with physical illness and that much of the time, we will appear to be amazingly fruitful at assisting with banishing mental distress. Yet, there are confinements, particularly with what can be accomplished utilizing self-hypnosis chronicles. A few things are better left for coordinated hypnotherapy, where there is that live association between people. If we don't accept, we can offer any genuine assistance or backing employing the mode of accounts; at that point, we won't produce them. Physical illnesses When physical illness is included, the circumstance is precarious, because most proofs of 'fixes' or abatements are recounted. It is notable and perceived by the standard clinical world that the invulnerable reaction, uneasiness, and the mental prosperity of any individual are closely connected. Along these lines, improving people's mental prosperity should enhance their physical well-being, which often appears to be the situation. Some trance inducers work specifically with, in critical condition, people utilizing hypno-analysis, which is a propelled type of hypnotherapy. There are a few cases, where after remedial mediation, a few patients endure and keep on enduring, long in the wake of having been proclaimed as 'past all expectation' by the standard clinical profession. Be that as it may, only one out of every odd time. The conviction behind this sort of work includes finding and settling the beginning reason for the self-destruct program that a few people accept exists in all in critical condition people. The theory – and it is just a speculation, though it is by all accounts demonstrated – is that discharging the 'caught' feeling, the constraint, permits the body to work precisely as it should, as a self-fixing machine. Additionally, on the off chance that it isn't self-evident, propelled hypnotherapy procedures, for example, hypnoanalysis, should ever be possible face to face. Hypnoanalysis is an extremely many-sided discipline that requires a lot of care and consideration. It isn't reasonable for everybody and is undoubtedly not something that should be possible by means of the vehicle of sound accounts.

One requires a progression of various sessions on self-hypnosis to receive its benefits, which may go up to at least six sessions. A few people come up short on the persistence or adequate supports basic for proceeding with the specified number of sessions. Numerous others believe that lone a solitary self-hypnosis session is sufficient to mend patients of their emotional disturbance and stress. This is a nonsensical conviction, and suspending such sessions would kill the impact of a solitary self-hypnosis session. One must teach the habit of rehearsing self-hypnosis consistently to make it solid. Patients must feel a sort of self-acknowledgment to make it work.

The whole procedure of self-hypnosis is gigantically relaxing and agreeable, which may make an impression in the minds of its patients that it isn't precisely valuable true to form. People may begin questioning its strength as there is nonattendance of any significant stun to the arrangement of the human body. This occurs as it is inherently associated with adjusting the thought forms through specific procedures. Along these lines, the change which happens, therefore, is acquainted with the patient by the sheer intensity of the mind and its astuteness and nothing else. One needs to be sufficiently handy to get a handle on how the change realized in one's framework is so ordinary and progressive that it is practically unnoticeable right away.

There exist a couple of people who become incredibly dependent on the system of self-hypnosis and start such courses for simple happiness and some new energy in their lives. They utilize self-hypnosis as an integral asset to escape from the real world, and this slowly turns into their habit. From that point, they become reliant on it for encountering typical delight.

CHAPTER TWENTY-ONE: GUIDE TO HYPNOSIS

The way to beat your feelings of trepidation could be as simple as benefiting as much as possible from reflection and positive affirmations. The best part is that you can do it from the solace of your home.

If you think hypnosis is something that occurs in front of an audience, complete with swinging pendants and people acting like chickens, well, we have news for you. While numerous people make this suspicion, it's a long way from the real world.

Hypnosis is less about what somebody does to you, and increasingly about how you can encourage your change. Envision it as a sort of reflection – with a scramble of personal improvement tossed in for good measure.

Regardless of whether you've always needed to overcome a dread that has been keeping you down or hoping to attempt an elective type of relaxation, there are numerous reasons why hypnosis could profit you. Everything necessary is a receptive outlook and a status to make a change for yourself. The best piece about it is that it's personal to you; there's no off-base or right way to go about self-hypnosis.

In any case, to assist you with a beginning, here is a five-advance guide stacked with convenient indications to assist you with finding a strategy that works for you:

1. Relax

The term hypnosis originates from the Greek word hupnos, signifying "rest." While self-hypnosis isn't about really falling asleep, we are progressively powerless to the proposal when we're relaxed.

Thus, locate a quiet situation where you aren't probably going to be upset and spot your telephone far out. Sit or rests in an agreeable position. Slow your breathing and let yourself relax all the more deeply with each breath.

The best piece about it is that it's personal to you; there's no off-base or right way to go about self-hypnosis.

2. Would it be advisable for me to close my eyes?

Trance inducers have different suppositions on this. Some believe that by keeping your eyes shut, it's simpler to shut out interruptions. This can help with focus and creative mind, permitting you to relax effectively and your unconscious mind to be increasingly open. In any case, if this feels awkward (or you wind up falling asleep!), simply leave your eyes open. The decision is yours.

3. Concentrate on the result you need

Push away restricting habits from your mind, and give a solid option of how you'd prefer to think or feel. Put firm confidence in what it is you need to accomplish. The significant thing is to envision yourself achieving your goals. For instance, if you need to quit any smoking pretense, envision yourself without cigarettes, fit and solid, and taking in outside air.

This helps put you in an "accomplishing" perspective that allows you to put stock in yourself and manifest energy in your life.

4. Practice affirmations

Utilize positive, simple explanations to fortify your thoughts. To effectively plant these thoughts in your unconscious, these announcements need to be certified, genuine, and simple – straightforward should as much as possible.

Use of "I," center around something specific, and always set up your announcements as current state realities. Keep in mind; this is you telling your unconscious that you can do it. To relieve stress at work, you may state, "I am relaxed at work." To defeat open talking nerves, you may say, "I am a sure speaker."

Focus on a couple of articulations and truly focus on them. Repeating this procedure is critical and will reinforce the association you have with this new way of reasoning.

5. Build up an everyday practice

Likewise, with anything, consistency is significant, as is standard practice. Discover a time in your day that you can resolve to, even if it's only for a couple of moments. At that point, stick to it.

Picture your future. How can it feel? Try not to stress over the procedure and moves it will make to arrive, simply have confidence in yourself and your capacity to make changes.

CHAPTER TWENTY-TWO: GREAT TIPS TO ELIMINATE YOUR CRAVINGS

Cravings are normal. Over half of individuals experience cravings all the time.

They assume a significant job in weight gain, food fixation, and binge eating.

Monitoring your cravings and their triggers makes them a lot simpler to maintain a strategic distance from. It likewise makes it significantly simpler to eat healthy and lose weight.

Following the guides below, for example, eating more protein, arranging your suppers, and rehearsing mindfulness, may permit you to assume responsibility for cravings attempting to dominate.

Dieting would be quite simple if it weren't for those cravings. Fortunately, there are numerous things you can do to make cravings a thing of the past. Step away from the snacks and look at these ten hints for beating your cravings.

1. Address Any Deficiencies

If you experience customary, serious cravings for particular foods, you might be experiencing a healthful inadequacy that your body is attempting to address. It is accepted that chocolate cravings can come from a magnesium insufficiency, while an absence of chromium in the diet can prompt sugar cravings. Keeping up healthy levels of zinc can likewise assist with directing your craving. Ensure you are eating a wide assortment of nutritious foods to address any insufficiencies in your diet.

2. Eat A Little Of What You Fancy

Ever discovered that your cravings deteriorated the harder you attempted to overlook them? A study distributed in the journal Appetite has suggested that numerous individuals long for the foods that they should endeavor to stand up to. As opposed to going immediately on your junk food dependence, having a tad bit of what you extravagant should assist with decreasing the impulse to binge on your preferred treats. You could have a go at following the 80/20 guideline, eating steadily 80 percent of the time and being less severe for the other 20 percent.

3. Get Active

Regardless of whether your cravings originate from

yearning, fatigue, or absence of inspiration, taking off for a run or going to the exercise center could help you not to yield. Exercise isn't just a great interruption from your cravings; a study has likewise discovered that oxygen consuming activity can assist with stifling your hunger. Moreover, getting dynamic will assist you with feeling great about your body, and you wouldn't have any desire to destroy all that difficult work with a junk food binge currently, would you?

4. Attempt Healthier Alternatives

Because you've chosen to eat soundly, that doesn't mean you can never snack again. As opposed to surrendering to your junk food cravings, take a stab at exploring different avenues for healthier alternatives, such as solidified yogurt or sorbet rather than frozen yogurt, prepared popcorn as opposed to crisps and yam wedges rather than fries.

5. Get Some Vanilla Scented Products

If you're battling to oppose sugar cravings, take a stab at putting resources into a vanilla-scented flame or deodorizer for your home or wearing a vanilla-scented fragrance to check cravings while in a hurry. A study found that utilizing vanilla-scented fixes on the rear of participants' hands significantly diminished their hunger for sweet foods and beverages. It is accepted this is because the smell of vanilla can assist with smothering sweet cravings.

6. Give Yourself A Happiness Boost

An Examination has discovered that eating starches, like pasta, bread, and potatoes, animate the creation of the 'happy hormone' serotonin in the cerebrum. This may clarify why a significant number of us pine for these 'comfort' foods when we're feeling down. To cut your cravings, attempt to discover healthier ways to give your serotonin levels a lift, for example, getting together with a companion, viewing a parody film, participating in an activity meeting, or smelling some uplifting fundamental oils, for example, neroli or lemon.

7. Unwind

Similarly, the same number of us enjoy comfort eating when we're feeling down; stress can likewise be a ground-breaking trigger for cravings.

Exploration from the University of Cincinnati has indicated that sodium in salt hinders the body's stress hormones, implying that cravings for salty foods could be your body's endeavor to manage stress. To defeat these cravings, attempt to avoid the things that cause you to stress as much as possible and make unwinding a customary part of your daily schedule. Locate a healthier way to manage stress when it happens, for example, working out, pondering, or talking through your issues with a companion.

8. Change Your Habits

As indicated by research results, your condition can be a ground-breaking trigger for food cravings. Possibly your partner setting off to the film with eating popcorn, for instance, or viewing your preferred TV show, makes you go after a snack. To exile habit-framed cravings, attempt to stay away from the conditions that trigger them. Take up a leisure activity that diminishes your TV time, or walk a different course to work so as not to pass by your preferred café. By staying away from specific spots or exercises, you can assist with executing those cravings.

9. Start Your Day With A Treat

While it might sound counterproductive, if your cravings are truly jumping on you, breakfast could be the ideal time to enjoy. Scientists from Tel Aviv University found that participants who had a 2500-kilojoule breakfast, which included sweet, lost an average of 40lbs (18.41kg) more than the individuals who had a little 1250-kilojoule one. This is thought to be because the digestion is increasingly productive in the first part of the day, and because surrendering to cravings first thing can assist with banishing them for the remainder of the day.

10. Get Enough Sleep

Scientists at the University of Chicago have discovered

that not getting enough rest influences our hunger controlling hormones, implying that we feel hungrier the following day and are additionally bound to ache for kilojoule-rich, high-sugar foods. Not just that, the absence of rest decreases self-control, implying that you are more averse to oppose those cravings. To help diminish your cravings, ensure you get at least seven hours of rest a night.

CHAPTER TWENTY-THREE: GUIDE MEDITATION TO LOSE WEIGHT FOR WOMEN

Diet and exercise might be key parts of weight loss for ladies, yet numerous different components assume a job.

Studies show that everything from rest quality to stress levels can majorly affect hunger, digestion, body weight, and belly fat.

Luckily, causing a couple of little changes in your everyday schedule can bring huge advantages with regard to weight loss.

1. Cut Down on Refined Carbs

Refined carbs experience broad handling, decreasing the measure of fiber and micronutrients in the last item.

These foods spike glucose levels, increase hunger, and are related to increased body weight and belly fat.

Consequently, it's ideal for restraining refined carbs like white bread, pasta, and prepackaged foods. Decide on entire grain items like oats, earthy colored rice, quinoa, buckwheat, and grain.

2. Add Resistance Training to Your Routine

Obstruction preparing manufactures muscle and increases perseverance.

It's particularly advantageous for ladies more than 50, as it increases the number of calories that your body burns very still. It likewise assists safeguard with boning mineral thickness to ensure against osteoporosis.

Lifting weights, utilizing rec center gear, or performing body-weight practices are a couple of basic ways to begin.

3. Drink More Water

Drinking more water is a simple and compelling way to promote weight loss with insignificant exertion.

One little study indicated that drinking 16.9 ounces (500 ml) of water briefly increased the number of calories burned by 30% after 30–40 minutes.

Studies likewise show that drinking water before a supper can increase weight loss and lessen the number of calories devoured by around 13%.

4. Eat More Protein

Protein foods like meat, poultry, seafood, eggs, dairy, and vegetables are a significant part of a healthy diet, particularly with regards to weight loss.

Studies note that following a high-protein diet can cut cravings, increase sentiments of totality, and lift digestion.

One little 12-week study additionally found that expanding protein admission by simply 15% decreased day by day calorie consumption by an average of 441 calories — bringing about 11 pounds (5 kg) of weight loss.

5. Set a Regular Sleep Schedule

Studies suggest that getting enough rest might be similarly as significant to losing weight as diet and exercise.

Different studies have related a lack of sleep with increased body weight and more elevated levels of ghrelin, the hormone liable for invigorating yearning.

Besides, one study in ladies demonstrated that getting at any rate seven hours of rest every night and generally improving rest quality increased the probability of weight loss success by 33%.

6. Accomplish More Cardio

Oxygen consuming activity, otherwise called cardio, increases your pulse to burn extra calories.

Studies show that adding more cardio to your routine can bring about significant weight loss — particularly when combined with a healthy diet.

For best outcomes, focus on in any event 20–40 minutes of cardio every day, or around 150–300 minutes out of each week.

7. Keep a Food Journal

Utilizing a food journal to follow what you eat is a simple way to consider yourself responsible and settle on healthier decisions.

It additionally makes the most of it simpler to calories, which can be a successful procedure for weight management.

Also, a food journal can assist you with adhering to your goals and may bring about greater long haul weight loss.

8. Top off on Fiber

Adding more fiber to your diet is a typical weight loss procedure to help moderate the discharging of your stomach and keep you feeling more full for more.

Without rolling out some other improvements to diet or lifestyle, expanding dietary fiber admission by 14 grams for every day has been related to a 10% decrease in calorie consumption and 4.2 pounds (1.9 kg) of weight loss over 3.8 months.

Natural products, vegetables, legumes, nuts, seeds, and entire grains are all great wellsprings of fiber that can be enjoyed as part of an appropriate diet.

9. Practice Mindful Eating

Mindful eating includes limiting outer interruptions during your dinner. Take a stab at eating slowly and concentrating on how your food tastes, looks, scents, and feels.

This training promotes healthier eating habits and is an amazing asset for expanding weight loss.

Studies show that eating slowly can upgrade sentiments of completion and may prompt significant decreases in everyday calorie consumption.

10. Snack Smarter

Choosing healthy, low-calorie snacks is a great way to lose weight and remain on target by limiting yearning levels between dinners.

Pick snacks that are high in protein and fiber to promote

completion and control cravings.

The entire organic product combined with nut margarine, veggies with hummus, or Greek yogurt with nuts are instances of nutritious snacks that can bolster permanent weight loss.

11. Discard the Diet

Although fad diets regularly guarantee snappy weight loss, they can accomplish more mischief than anything about your waistline and your well-being.

For instance, one study in school ladies demonstrated that killing certain foods from their diet increased cravings and overeating.

Fad diets can likewise promote unhealthy eating habits and lead to yo-yo dieting, the two of which are inconvenient to long haul weight loss.

12. Press in More Steps

When you're in a hurry and incapable of fitting in a full exercise, pressing more strides into your day is a simple way to burn extra calories and increase weight loss.

Indeed, it's evaluated that non-workout related action may represent half of the calories your body burns for the duration of the day.

Using the stairwell rather than the lift, stopping further

from the entryway, or going for a stroll during your mid-day break are a couple of straightforward techniques to knock up your absolute number of steps and burn more calories.

13. Set Attainable Goals

Defining SMART goals can make it simpler to reach your weight loss goals while also setting you up for success.

Shrewd goals ought to be specific, quantifiable, attainable, applicable, and time-bound. They should consider you responsible and spread out an arrangement for how to arrive at your goals.

For instance, rather than essentially defining a goal to lose 10 pounds, set a goal to lose 10 pounds in 3 months by keeping a food journal, heading off to the exercise center three times for every week, and adding a serving of vegetables to every supper.

14. Monitor Stress

A few studies suggest that increased stress levels can add to a greater danger of weight gain after some time.

Stress may likewise change eating examples and add to issues like overeating and gorging.

Working out, tuning in to music, rehearsing yoga,

journaling, and conversing with companions or family are a few simple and powerful ways to bring down stress levels.

15. Attempt HIIT

High-power spans preparation, otherwise called HIIT, sets extraordinary development eruptions with brief recuperation periods to help keep your pulse raised.

Trading cardio for HIIT a couple of times for every week would amp be able to up weight loss.

HIIT can decrease belly fat, increase weight loss, and appear to burn more calories than different exercises, for example, biking and running.

16. Use Smaller Plates

Changing to a littler plate size may help promote parcel control, supporting weight loss.

Although research stays restricted and conflicting, one study indicated that participants who used a littler plate ate less and felt more fulfilled than those who used a typical size plate.

Utilizing a little plate can likewise restrain your bit size, which can decrease your danger of overeating and hold calorie utilization under wraps.

17. Take a Probiotic Supplement

Probiotics are a sort of gainful microscopic organisms that can be devoured through food or enhancements to assist support with gutting well-being.

Studies show that probiotics can promote weight loss by expanding the discharge of fat and changing hormone levels to diminish craving.

In particular, Lactobacillus gasseri is a strain of probiotic that is particularly compelling. Studies show that it can assist a decrease in bellying fat and, generally speaking, body weight.

18. Practice Yoga

Studies show that rehearsing yoga can help prevent weight gain and increase fat burning.

Yoga can likewise decrease stress levels and tension — the two of which might be attached to passionate eating.

Moreover, rehearsing yoga has been appeared to lessen binge eating and prevent distraction with food to help healthy eating practices.

19. Bite Slower

Putting forth a cognizant attempt to bite slowly and altogether can assist an increase with weighting loss by eliminating the measure of food you eat.

One study indicated that biting 50 times for each chomp significantly decreased calorie consumption contrasted with biting 15 times for each nibble.

Another study demonstrated that biting food either 150% or 200% more than ordinary decreased food admission by 9.5% and 14.8%, individually.

20. Eat a Healthy Breakfast

Getting a charge out of a nutritious breakfast before anything else can help start your day off on the correct foot and keep you feeling full until your next dinner.

Studies locate that adhering to a standard eating example might be connected to a diminished danger of binge eating.

Eating a high-protein breakfast has been appeared to decrease levels of the yearning advancing hormone ghrelin. This can help monitor craving and appetite.

21. Analysis With Intermittent Fasting

Intermittent fasting includes switching back and forth among eating and fasting for a specific window of time every day. Times of fasting commonly last 14–24 hours.

Intermittent fasting is thought to be as successful as slicing calories with regards to weight loss.

It might likewise help upgrade digestion by expanding

the quantity of calories burned very still.

22. Breaking point Processed Foods

Processed foods are normally high in calories, sugar, and sodium, yet they are low in significant supplements like protein, fiber, and micronutrients.

Studies show that devouring progressively processed foods is related to the abundance of body weight — particularly among ladies.

In this way, it's ideal to restrict your admission of processed foods and decide on whole foods, for example, natural products, vegetables, healthy fats, lean proteins, entire grains, and vegetables.

23. Cut Back on Added Sugar

Included sugar is a significant supporter of weight gain and genuine medical problems, for example, diabetes and coronary illness.

Foods high in included sugar are stacked with extra calories yet ailing in the nutrients, minerals, fiber, and protein that your body needs to flourish.

Therefore, it's ideal to limit your admission of sweet foods like pop, treats, organic product juice, sports beverages, and desserts to help promote weight loss and improve by and large well-being.

MORE TIPS

The pants don't lie. You realized you let yourself go a smidgen, and subsequent to discarding the dumb washroom scale because it said you were (embed warning number here), you went for the genuine test — slipping on your preferred pants. Not having the option to pull your jeans past your thighs sure discloses to you something. If you're at a loss with regards to how to start, here's a simple, direct, 11-advance manual for losing weight.

Calories every day: Losing weight is tied in with creating a calorie deficiency. One pound rises to 3,500 calories, which separates to 500 calories per day. Do a combo of activity and slicing calories to arrive at 500, and you'll lose a pound a week. You can meet with a nutritionist or your primary care physician to locate an increasingly specific day by day calorie tally, yet don't plunge underneath 1,200 as it will hinder your digestion.

Follow along: Monitor your calories as precisely as could be expected under the circumstances. Look into calorie sums, and record them in a food journal, or use a weight-loss application. Everything you put in your mouth gets recorded — indeed, even that bunch of M&M's you got off your collaborator's work area! It may not appear a lot, yet at 70 calories, those little snacks will include. At that point, gauge yourself on more than one occasion per week to monitor your advancement.

Measure and repeat: Have estimating cups, spoons, and food scales available to gauge the right parts. Eyeballing a cup of grain isn't exactly exact, and you'd be shocked that it is so natural to overestimate your eagerness. In the initial hardly any months, you'll have to gauge everything; from the milk, you fill that bowl of oat to the dressing; you sprinkle on your serving of mixed greens. Sooner or later, you'll become acquainted with what right bits resemble.

Eat five times per day: In request to prevent that hungry inclination that drives us to overeat, plan on eating three suppers and two snacks per day, timing them, so you eat each a few hours. Here's an example plan:

- 7 a.m. — Breakfast
- 9:30 a.m. — Snack
- 12:30 p.m. — Lunch
- 3:30 p.m. — Snack
- 6:30 p.m. — Dinner

Try not to skip dinners or snacks to spare calories since it'll hinder your digestion and cause weight gain. If you're up late, appreciate a snack after supper, however, make certain to complete it, in any event, an hour or two preceding bed, so stomach related problems don't keep you up — getting enough rest will assist you with losing weight.

What to eat: Whenever you grub, make certain to incorporate protein to fulfill your craving, fiber to top you off, and healthy carbs to support your energy. Breakfast, lunch, and supper can be somewhere in the range of 300 and 500 calories each, and the two snacks 150 each. Separate them to meet your requirements, yet you may need your midday dinner to be the most elevated to guarantee you have sufficient opportunity to burn off those calories.

Additional calories: Find basic ways to cut calories, regardless of whether it's trading your daily Coke for water, utilizing one cut of cheddar on your sandwich rather than two, subbing spaghetti squash for pasta, or picking a turkey patty rather than a hamburger.

Plan ahead: Dealing with hunger is the most exceedingly awful part about attempting to lose weight, to prevent those aches from pushing you to snatch the closest treat, plan out your suppers and snacks early. Work out what you'll be eating for the whole week, and you'll be even increasingly successful if you pack and mark foods every day.

Get going: Diet is one part of the weight-loss puzzle, and the other part is working out. So as to burn calories to decrease your general body fat, incorporate an hour of heart-siphoning exercise five times per week. A relaxed stroll around the square sadly isn't sufficient. We're talking, running, biking, swimming, and high-power classes for cardio, quality preparing to manufacture fat-burning muscles, and extending to keep those muscles flexible and to prevent injury. Here's an hour-long exercise to kick you off that consolidates every one of the three.

Set little goals and commend them: Losing weight is a long excursion, so it's useful to set littler goals en route to your large goal. Find healthy ways to praise those achievements, such as a pedicure after ten exercises or a charming exercise top in the wake of losing five pounds.

Go to some extreme acknowledge: The first is that diets aren't the appropriate response. There is no handy solution diet and nobody food you can or can't eat with mysterious thinning powers. Anything that sounds excessively prohibitive or not healthfully solid isn't the way to go. Discover a way of eating that can be continued for the remainder of your life, where you eat healthy more often than not and take into account periodic lavish expenditures. The subsequent acknowledgment is that you can't return to your old habits once the weight liquefies away. If you gained weight biting on about six doughnuts every morning, you could wager your sweet new buns that you'll gain the weight back if you head to that bread shop once the scale says what you need it to.

About Your Diet

Be understandable and recall why you're doing it: Just

as those pounds slowly crawled on, losing weight the correct way requires some investment, which means dropping about a pound or two per week. Practice tolerance, delighting in each pound lost, and when you want to surrender to that second cupcake at your companion's birthday party, have one hugely close to home explanation you need to lose weight that resounds solid and keeps you propelled regardless. Thinking "I need to be there for my family" makes certain to be more compelling than "I need to glance great in my pants."

CHAPTER TWENTY-FOUR: AFFIRMATIONS FOR WEIGHT LOSS FOR WOMEN

We, as a whole, have designs running inside our psyche mind, which start at an early age. We're vigorously impacted by our loved ones, just as our condition. If you were repeatedly given chocolate as a youngster to make you quit crying, odds are you have a profoundly attached grapple to chocolate, and partner it with causing you to feel better when you feel upset in your grown-up life.

By and large, the habits we structure at an early age are advantageous to us because they ensure us and make us special; however, some can be adverse to our prosperity and cause us to self-sabotage (i.e., enthusiastic eating). Affirmations are a great way to send positive messages to your oblivious mind with the goal that you begin to think and act in a more pleasant way towards yourself.

Going from negative self converse with self-esteem doesn't occur without any forethought.

What is an affirmation?

For a positive affirmation to be successful, determine first the sort of change you need to make, for example, a result, goal, or mindset that you need to create.

Scientific studies affirm that utilizing affirmations can "rework" your cerebrum and help you roll out positive improvements in your life.

A few people accept that it takes a few weeks of repeating an individual affirmation before you get results, so attempt to keep on saying your constructive affirmation day by day for a month.

From the outset, you'll have to settle on a cognizant choice to repeat your affirmations.

Notwithstanding, after some time, they will begin to supplant the negative thoughts that will assume control over when you aren't checking your thoughts.

Step by step instructions to use everyday affirmations for ladies

Here are the means to fortify female affirmations in your mind, so it turns into your characteristic way of reasoning or acting:

Stage 1: Keep an affirmation journal, and record the affirmation you are taking a shot at. Concentrate on each affirmation in turn.

Stage 2: Speak the affirmation so anyone can hear, before a mirror, preferably, three times every day for around five minutes.

You can do this while preparing toward the beginning of the day or before bed. In the day, discover a time previously or after lunch to repeat your affirmation before a mirror.

Stage 3: Visualize that the affirmation is now valid for you. See yourself carrying on and thinking in the way portrayed in the affirmation.

Going about just as the affirmation is as of now genuine gives you the psychological capacity to make it genuine.

Make a new beginning with constructive reasoning and trust in the incredible asset of individual affirmations.

Here is a rundown of uplifting, positive affirmation models for ladies that you can begin utilizing today.

Pick one individual affirmation that addresses you as a lady. At that point, list the changes you need to make in your self-observations and individual goals.

Weight loss is one of the most widely recognized goals or New Year's goals. Regardless of whether your explanation is better wellbeing or you need to be more joyful with your physical appearance and feel better in your own skin, weight loss is conceivable and can be both simple and fun!

Gaining extra pounds is simpler than losing them. Be that as it may, if you reprogram your mind and have a perfectly clear vision of the amount you need to gauge, accomplishing your fantasy weight will be simpler than you at any point thought.

It is ideal to begin with affirmations that are increasingly sensible and reachable. A superior one in this circumstance is, "I'm getting more slender consistently!" By making your affirmations increasingly practical, they will become a reality sooner. Separate your weight loss goals and affirmations in little, feasible augmentations. You need to fabricate success rapidly as that will gather the positive energy and speed for more success!

At the point when you start to use affirmations for weight loss, you may see obstruction coming up for you very quickly. This is not out of the ordinary. A great many people surrender as of now. This obstruction is the basic part of your mind making statements like, "This is moronic." "This will never work." Or "You'll never lose this weight, and so on." This is likewise the voice of the saboteur within you. This is the part of you that wouldn't like to change. It has a personal stake in keeping you fat.

At the point when this opposition comes up, use one of the accompanying affirmations:

- I will change.

- I can do this.
- I have the ability to change my life.
- Indeed, I can!

Repeat these habitually for the duration of the day until you feel less obstruction. Keep in mind, your weight and overeating have been serving you somehow or another. It has been filling a void or addressing some need in your life. Alongside doing affirmations and perceptions, you should discover what that void or need is and locate a healthier, positive way of filling it. If you don't, you will rapidly slip by again into your old ruinous practices. This is one of the fundamental reasons why diets come up short.

Affirmations for Losing Weight and Getting Healthy

Affirmations are ground-breaking to use when you are going into circumstances that cause you to overeat. If you're at an eatery or party where you are enticed by the food you can repeatedly say one of the accompanying affirmations:

- I eat just what I need.
- I decide to eat healthy foods.
- I decide to remain on target.
- I am focused on my goals.

- I easily remain on target.
- I eat foods that help my new weight.
- I eat like a flimsy individual.

Repeating affirmations at these times will keep you focused and on target to meet your weight loss goals.

Utilizing affirmations will assist you with beginning self-supporting yourself. If you beat yourself up about your weight or tear down your body, use affirmations. If, when glancing in the mirror, you make statements like, "You have such thunder thighs." "Take a gander at that cellulite." "I despise my butt, stomach, body, and so forth." Choose to state positive affirmations like this:

- I am much obliged to you for serving me.
- I am getting more grounded and slimmer consistently.
- I treat my body with love and thoughtfulness.
- My body is the sanctuary of my soul.

We begin to accept what we are stating, and we put our words vigorously.

1. I have the ability to create change.

2. I am accountable for how I feel, and today I am picking satisfaction.

3. I can, and I will.

4. I put stock in the individual I am turning out to be.

5. I am giving a valiant effort, and that is always enough.

6. I have the ability to change my thoughts in a second.

7. I rest in satisfaction when I rest, realizing everything is great in my reality.

8. By permitting myself to be upbeat, I move others to be glad too.

9. Mistakes and difficulties are venturing stones to my success because I gain from them.

10. I know precisely what I have to do to make progress.

11. I embrace the here and now and am certain of things to come.

12. I favor of myself and love myself profoundly and totally.

Glad Woman

13. I confide in myself and realize my inward astuteness is my best guide.

14. I decide to be glad for myself.

15. With each breath out, I discharge stress in my body.

16. My body is mending, and I feel much improved and better each day.

17. I am grounded in the experience of the current second.

18. I watch my thoughts and activities without making a decision about them.

19. Life is going on at this time.

20. I acknowledge and grasp all encounters, even undesirable ones.

21. I am better than negative thoughts and low activities.

22. Creative energy surges through me and leads me to new and splendid thoughts.

23. Satisfaction is my decision.

24. I am honored with a staggering family and great companions.

25. I am a powerhouse, and I am indestructible.

Keep in mind, each grievance that you state to yourself is a negative affirmation of something you are troubled about in your life.

At whatever point you blow up, you're telling the universe that you need more anger. At whatever point you feel like a casualty, you're advising the universe that you need to be in a casualty job.

If you accept life isn't giving you what you want or need, you will never have the advantages that life offers to other people — until you adjust your mindset.

These constructive affirmations for ladies will assist you with traversing your intense days and accomplish your goals for certainty, self-awareness, and success.

Keep in mind, the more you support and fuel your internal identity, the more engaged you will feel, and the more inspired you will be to overcome the days in front of you.

CHAPTER TWENTY-FIVE: EAT HEALTHY WITH SUBLIMINAL HYPNOSIS

How frequently have you begun a weight loss program just to encounter the baffling truth of not having the option to remain with it?

For instance, intentionally, you might be determined to eat healthy foods and dodge inexpensive fatty food and void calories. But when you pass by the calorie-loaded treats, you simply yield, time after time.

Why?

That is because your inner mind programmed practices are more grounded than any self-control you may assemble.

As you may know, programmed practices are followed up on from your inner mind, which is altogether liable for your lingering and negative self-talk.

Stuff like, I'll simply have this bit of cake today, tomorrow I'll eat healthy or, I'll begin practicing one week from now or, No matter what I do, I'm not ready to lose weight without any end in sight.

Anguishing, right?

That is the place a subliminal program comes to help.

Incredibly, the unintelligible subliminal entrancing guidelines sidestep the systematic channel of your cognizant mind and reach your inner mind straightforwardly, where genuine change happens.

With normal use, subliminals help you to reprogram your inner mind tenderly.

You need to realize the advantages you get from the specific spellbinding directions of a subliminal weight loss program, isn't that so?

Some of them are:

- Increased metabolic rate and physical energy
- No more food cravings, desserts or junk food cravings
- Decreased by and large hunger
- Obtained preference for healthy foods
- The specific mindset of a thin and fit individual
- Not any more self-subverting thoughts and practices
- Greatly increased inspiration and self-assurance.
- Simply consider it.

The unintelligible messages in the Subliminal Weight Loss program change profound seated habits; accordingly, you quit being tormented by food cravings and enthusiastic eating. Over time, utilizing this sort of self spellbinding for weight loss, the extra pounds fall away, permitting you to arrive at your optimal weight effortlessly – and save it for good.

What Exactly are Subliminal Weight Loss Messages?

If you've at any point pondered about it, entrancing is tied in with disassembling restricting convictions and reprogramming your mind for all the more engaging ones so healthy practices become natural to you.

In any case, if you attempted ordinary self spellbinding for weight loss, you know how sometimes your cognizant mind will, in general, oppose the perceptible messages, making them incapable, best case scenario, disappointing even from a pessimistic standpoint, correct?

That is because your cognizant mind (so stuck in a rut) dismisses direct verbal messages sifting through the specific suggestions intended to revise your unhelpful examples of conduct. Therefore, they never arrive at your inner mind, where your programmed convictions and practices live.

It's actual; you're infrequently mindful of your psyche

mind. It is much the same as that shrouded away underneath the surface, the greater part of a chunk of ice.

In all honesty, this much bigger part of your mind is liable for your preferences, profound seated convictions, habits, and programmed examples of conduct when confronted with different circumstances and difficulties.

While your psyche is in control to keep you alive no matter what, it carries out this responsibility depending on what has worked in the past for you, paying little mind to how well it functions for you NOW.

As fantastic as it might appear, your inner mind can't understand HOW something functions – it just uses anything it goes over – that is, IF it isn't sifted through by your cognizant mind.

It sounds practically crazy, isn't that right?

To fathom this, a subliminal program contains verbal suggestions recorded at a higher sound recurrence, beneath your hearing level and ordinary cognizant mindfulness, on a quiet or loosening up music foundation. The quiet, subliminal content detours your cognizant mind and effectively arrives at your inner mind along these lines.

Here, at your inner mind level, the spellbinding guidelines break down any obsolete, adapted convictions about yourself and your body that are keeping you away from your present goals. After some time, you easily discharge any passionate examples that have sabotaged your best goals previously.

Simultaneously, the subliminal suggestions engrave another arrangement of self-enabling convictions that realize a perpetual change in your life. Specific trigger words and expressions grapple in your inner mind a "being healthy, cut and conditioned" mindset, which bolsters consequently any weight loss or work out regime.

With standard tuning in, your disposition towards healthy eating and being dynamic changes totally in a couple of short weeks. As this occurs (at the rear of your mind, in a manner of speaking), you become so determined that nothing can stop you.

You naturally settle on healthy decisions around food, turning out to be simply turned into a typical part of your life. You get the opportunity to appreciate it.

At that point, when you accomplish your goal, this enabled mindset keeps you at your optimal weight easily.

Simply take a load off for 30 minutes every day, and let your inner mind be reprogrammed with healthy eating habits naturally.

- You will lose every one of your cravings for food that isn't helpful to you.

- Your energy levels will rise, and you will feel great.
- Eliminate that slow resting state that you constantly walk around in.
- Never need to stress over diabetes, coronary illness, or elevated cholesterol again.
- Automatically build up the self-discipline to eat healthy food and love it.
- Junk food will have no intrigue to you any longer.
- You will consequently float towards healthy life-upgrading foods.
- Never diet again, let your psyche mind change the way you take a gander at food until the end of time.
- I hunger for healthy, nutritious food.
- I eat for wellbeing.
- As I lose weight, I keep it off.
- Eating healthy food is typical for me.
- Eating healthy is normal for me.
- Consistently I love my body to an ever-increasing extent.
- Feeling fit is astounding.
- I always stick to eating a healthy diet.

- I am constantly and securely softening fat from my body.
- I am thankful for my weight loss success.
- I purchase just unprocessed, healthy food.
- I can feel my muscles getting more grounded.
- I can abandon snacking.
- I pick foods deliberately.
- I have more energy.
- I feel better each day.
- I decide to be slim and fit.
- I decide to imagine myself flimsy and fit today.
- I intentionally pick what I put into my mouth.
- I constantly find physical exercises I appreciate.
- I have the right to appreciate eating refreshingly.
- I have the right to lose weight securely and quickly, and I do.
- I have the right to set aside the effort to practice normally.
- I effectively discharge my craving for unhealthy foods.
- I eat a reasonable diet.
- I eat for wellbeing.
- I eat healthy food consistently.

- I eat heaps of vegetables and servings of mixed greens.
- I eat little food divides.
- I quit eating before I am full.
- I appreciate taking a gander at myself in the mirror.
- I feel hunger just when my body needs food.
- I feel myself turning out to be lighter every day.
- I feel exceptionally slim and happy today and always.
- I feel extremely slim today and always.
- I have a healthy relationship with food.
- I have chosen to be dainty.
- I have no preference for unhealthy food.
- I like looking for food that is beneficial to me.
- I love myself now, and as I lose weight.
- I love serving of mixed greens.
- I love vegetables.
- I no longer ache for cheap food.
- I just eat enough food to evacuate my craving.
- I just eat foods that are beneficial to me.
- I just eat healthy food.
- I possibly eat when I am eager.

- I prefer Nutritious foods.
- I prefer to eat vegetables and natural products.
- I no longer want salt or sugar.
- I discharge any sentiments of being fat or unfit.
- I discharge abundance weight from all parts of my body.
- I discharge overabundance weight rapidly and without any problem.
- It's simpler to lose weight now that I have positive energy.
- It's simple for me to discover healthy snacks that I love.
- It's anything but difficult to add new leafy foods to my diet.
- It's energizing to watch my body regaining its more slender shape.
- It's alright to lose weight rapidly.
- I am in charge of what I eat.
- I am roused to get fit and healthy at this point.
- I am presently liberated from the longing to snack.
- My craving effectively remains leveled out always.
- My hunger is diminishing every day.

- I eat for wellbeing.
- My body appreciates losing weight and does it well overall.
- My body promptly acknowledges healthy food and drink.
- My body holds immaculate extents while losing weight.
- My hips and thighs become littler every day.
- My mind and body convey better each day.
- My stomach and midsection keep on contracting day by day.
- My weight is rapidly coming back to its optimal numbers.
- Today I can feel my fat liquefying away.
- Today and for the remainder of my life, I am fit.
- Today is my opportunity to be healthy.
- What I put in my mouth is up to me.
- I am healthy.

CHAPTER TWENTY-SIX: - POSITIVE THINKING AFFIRMATIONS

Positive affirmations for success are significant, and when they are done reliably and appropriately, they can prevent you from thinking negativity and undermining yourself. They can help you reprogram your mind and help you eliminate your restricting convictions.

Success is an internal mind game; if you can see yourself as somebody who achieves anything they set their mind to, chances are you will become that individual.

Positive affirmations are the correspondence between the conscious thought part of the mind and the inner mind activity part of the mind. We use positive affirmations for success or negative affirmations every day without even pondering it.

Many affirmations are negative, which, for the most part, prompts low confidence, awful dynamic, and a negative demeanor. You can assume control over it and perform what is called self-entrancing to quiet and control your mind. On the other hand, you can utilize one of the most effortless and least expensive ways to improve your mind and prosperity, which is the use of positive affirmations for success.

The Importance of Positive Affirmations

The main reason many people do not arrive at their maximum capacity is because they fail to take action to arrive at their goals and dreams. They proceed to hold on to the restricting beliefs that their folks have ingrained in them.

With the goal for you to accomplish your goals and have the courage to continue pushing ahead, you must work on saying positive affirmations for success consistently.

Each time you use positive affirmations for success, it sends a positive message to your inner mind. A decent arrangement of positive affirmations for success can help welcome riches, great wellbeing, and overhauled status in your life.

10 Positive Affirmations for Success

Positive affirmations for success can give us the correct mentality even under unexpected difficult conditions. Useful tidbits are out there to give us a head start, and we should simply use it much to our advantage.

So here they are, change your life with these ten affirmations for success:

1. My body is healthy; my mind is splendid; my spirit is peaceful

A healthy body begins with a healthy mind and soul. If either experiences negative feelings, the others will be influenced.

The number one cause of health or disease is you. You can also remove and revoke all permission that you have given consciously, subconsciously, to all the ills of the world because you share that pain.

You are conquering your sickness and defeating it consistently every day through positive affirmations.

2. I trust I can do anything

You need to say this to yourself every day. Because this is something that is so important for counseling yourself to stay encouraged.

By saying this, you can do anything and everything that you set your attention to.

3. Everything that is going on now is going on for my definitive great

There are no casualties, no mishaps, and no fortuitous events EVER. They just don't exist in this reality as you and others will just draw in what you and they are parts of.

In all seriousness occurs for an explanation and in

immaculate synchronicity.

4. I am the engineer of my life; I manufactured its establishment and picked its substance

Affirmation is something that you should reveal to yourself when you get up each morning. Each new day offers a new beginning and affects others around you. You can make anything of that day that you like because you are the engineer of your own life.

If you start your day with a positive affirmation of thoughts and feelings, it will change your day into something mind-boggling. Works unfailingly!

5. I excuse the individuals who have hurt me from quite a while ago and peacefully detach from them

That doesn't mean you overlook what they did, yet you find a sense of contentment with what they did and the exercises served.

Your solidarity to pardon is the thing that permits you to push ahead, and your response to any experience is autonomous of what others consider you.

6. My capacity to vanquish my difficulties is boundless; my capability to succeed is limitless

Straightforward, you have no restrictions yet those you

place on yourself.

What sort of life do you need? What is stopping you? What hindrances would you say you are forcing on yourself?

This positive affirmation will assist you with tending to the entirety of the limits.

7. Today, I forsake my old habits and take up new positive ones

Understand that any difficult time is just a short phase of life. This also will go alongside your old habits as you take in the new.

You are completely adjusting to being with creative energy, which surges through you and leads you to new and splendid thoughts and the mindset that allows that energy to stream.

8. I can accomplish greatness

One of the most remarkable affirmations is to let yourself know every day that you can accomplish all the greatness in life. Concentrate on your vision and dreams. At that point, connect the feeling to that vision.

By advising this positive affirmation to yourself and accepting that you can accomplish greatness, you enable yourself to create the life you want.

9. Today, I am overflowing with energy and flooding with satisfaction

Delight begins from within, not from outside of yourself. It additionally begins when you rise.

So make it a habit to repeat positive proclamations to yourself the first thing.

10. I love and accept myself for who I am

Self-esteem is intended to be the most perfect and most unique type of love. At the point when you love yourself, you consequently begin acknowledging and regarding yourself.

If you have certainty and pride in what you do, you will start to rethink yourself and be encouraged and enlivened to improve things with affirmations for success.

Affirmations to change your life

- I am the designer of my life; I construct its establishment and pick its substance.
- Today, I am overflowing with energy and flooding with delight.
- My body is healthy; my mind is splendid; my spirit is peaceful.

- I am better than negative thoughts and low activities.
- I have been given unlimited abilities, which I start to use today.
- I pardon the individuals who have hurt me from quite a while ago and peacefully detach from them.
- A stream of sympathy washes away my anger and replaces it with love.
- I am guided in all my means by Spirit, who drives me towards what I should know and do.
- (If you're hitched) My marriage is getting more grounded, further, and progressively stable every day.
- I have the characteristics that should have been very successful.
- (For entrepreneurs) My business is developing, extending, and flourishing.
- Creative energy surges through me and leads me to new and splendid thoughts.
- Happiness is a decision. I base my satisfaction on my own achievements and the favors I've been given.

- My capacity to vanquish my difficulties is boundless; my capability to succeed is interminable.
- (For the jobless individuals), I have the right to be utilized and paid well for my time, endeavors, and thoughts. Every day, I am closer to securing the ideal position for me.
- I am courageous, and I go to bat for myself.
- My thoughts are loaded up with energy, and my life is plentiful with thriving.
- Today, I forsake my old habits and take up new, progressively positive ones.
- Many individuals admire me and perceive my value; I am respected.
- I am honored with an unimaginable family and brilliant companions.
- I recognize my self-esteem; my certainty is taking off.
- Everything that is going on now is going on for my definitive great.
- I am a powerhouse; I am indestructible.
- Though these times are difficult, they are just a short phase of life.

- My future is a perfect projection of what I imagine now.
- My endeavors are being upheld by the universe; my fantasies manifest into reality before my eyes.
- (For the single individuals) The ideal partner for me is coming into my life sooner than I anticipated.
- I transmit excellence, appeal, and beauty.
- I am conquering my ailment; I am defeating it consistently every day.
- My deterrents are moving out of my way; my way is cut towards greatness.
- I wake up today with quality in my heart and clarity in my mind.
- My feelings of trepidation of tomorrow are just liquefying away.
- I am content with every one of that has occurred, is going on, and will occur.
- My inclination is Divine; I am an otherworldly being.
- My life is simply starting.
- I create a protected and secure space for myself in any place I am.

- I allow myself to make the right decision for me.
- I am positive about my capacity to [fill in the blank].
- I use my time and gifts to help other people [fill in the blank].
- What I love about myself is my capacity to [fill in the blank].
- I feel pleased with myself when I [fill in the blank].
- I give myself space to develop and learn.
- I permit myself to be who I am without judgment.
- I tune in to my instinct and trust my inward guide.
- I acknowledge my feelings and let them fill their need.
- I give myself the consideration and consideration that I merit.
- My drive and aspiration permit me to accomplish my goals.
- I offer my abilities with the world by [fill in the blank].
- I am acceptable at helping other people to [fill in the blank].

- I am always headed in the correct way.
- I trust that I am in the correct way.
- I am creatively roused by my general surroundings.
- My mind is loaded with splendid thoughts.
- I put my energy into things that matter to me.
- I confide in myself to settle on the correct choice.
- I am getting closer to my actual self consistently.

- I appreciate that there are people in my life who [fill in the blank].
- I am taking in important exercises from myself consistently.
- I am content with who I am as an individual.
- I have any kind of effect on the planet by essentially existing in it.

CHAPTER TWENTY-SEVEN: AFFIRMATIONS TO GREATLY IMPROVE YOUR LIFESTYLE

The flood of love in our way of life can't be coordinated, I concede, yet it is seldom about showing a youngster to be sure and sure about life, or about having confidence in their capacities to settle on keen decisions or to follow a fantasy. It is tied in with ensuring they keep the guidelines, with compliance always being the gauge over all things.

If you didn't grow up being told exactly how extraordinary and uncommon you are, how competent you are of everything you need to turn out to be, that it is so ordinary to have dreams outside of the standard, and the amount you matter to this world, this blog entry is for you, sweetheart!

If you need to be glad and successful in your own life, a constructive, furious, pleased and cheerful individual without disgrace, figure out how to be sure, and love and favor of yourself with these guided affirmation soundtracks. Use them day by day, and you'll bring about your temperaments and satisfaction levels in 7 days at the most recent.

Affirmations work best in the PRESENT tense, similarly as you see beneath, and when you state them intentionally and preferably uproariously (if the condition licenses!). Additionally, it assists with receiving positive BELIEVING just as positive THINKING as you grasp these words in the circumstances that emerge in your life.

At the point when you feel desolate and tragic:

- I feel the love of the individuals who are not genuinely around me.
- I enjoy my own isolation.
- I am too enormous a gift to this world to have self-sympathy.
- I love and endorse myself.
- At the point when you feel terrified (without your wellbeing being in danger):
- I center around breathing and establishing myself.
- Following my instinct and my heart keeps me free from any danger.
- I settle on the correct decisions without fail.
- I draw from my inward quality and light.
- I confide in myself.
- At the point when you feel insignificant:

- I am a remarkable offspring of this world.
- I have as much splendor to offer the world as anyone else.
- I matter and what I bring to the table this world likewise matters.
- I might be one out of 7 billion, yet I am additionally one out of 7 billion.
- At the point when you are anxious or apprehensive:
- I confide in my inward astuteness and instinct.
- I breathe in tranquility and breathe out anxiety.
- This circumstance works out for my most elevated great.
- Brilliant things unfurl before me.
- At the point when you are furious:
- I excuse myself for all the mistakes I have made.
- I let go of my anger so I can see clearly.
- I acknowledge the obligation if my anger has harmed anybody.
- I supplant my anger with comprehension and sympathy.
- I offer an expression of remorse to those influenced by my anger.

- At the point when you feel sad and pushed beyond your limits:
- I may not comprehend the positive qualities in this circumstance, yet it is there.
- I gather up more expectations and courage from somewhere inside me.
- I decide to discover cheerful and hopeful ways to take a gander at this.
- I compassionately request help and direction if I can't see a superior way.
- I refuse to surrender because I haven't attempted every single imaginable way.
- I release old habits that are constraining my latent capacity.
- I appreciate eating healthy food.
- My food decisions and my weight don't characterize who I am.
- I decide to relinquish foolish examples that don't serve me.
- My body is entire and full.
- Although I can't see all that is in front of me, I can make the following stride.
- I can just discover by attempting.

- I am solid and quiet.
- My health is an interest in my life.
- Today I'm deciding to be daring.
- I confide in my own procedure.
- My body is my home, and I'm going to deal with it.
- I pick life.
- I don't have to exercise to merit food.
- I treat my body with deference.
- My body needs me to feed it with the goal that I can carry on with a happy life.
- How I feel about myself has nothing to do about what I eat or don't eat.
- Today I allow myself to be greater than my feelings of dread.
- Dread is just an inclination; it can't keep me down.
- Affirmations to quit dieting and tallying calories
- I will come out of this recuperating procedure, healthier and more astute.
- Life is too short to even think about counting calories.
- I'm tallying the recollections, not the calories.

- My life is driven by my aim and motivation, not calories.
- I won't permit calories to disrupt the general flow of a glad life.
- A goal weight is an excessive number and doesn't talk about my health.
- You no longer control me, calories, I am free.
- I eat for energy and sustenance.
- Food isn't the adversary. It is supporting and recuperating.
- How I feel about myself has nothing to do about what I eat or don't eat.
- I confide during the time spent recuperation.
- I treat my body with deference.
- Affirmations to develop positive body image
- I am OK.
- I feed my body healthy, supporting food, and give it healthy sustaining exercise because it has the right to be dealt with.
- My mind is my hottest body part.
- I can have a decent day even when I am not happy in my body.

- I am available to and acknowledge the sentiment of being sufficient simply the way I am.
- I let go of negative thoughts and travel through life in bliss.
- I acknowledge my body and feel good in my skin.
- My body is beautiful; I will regard and care for it.
- There is nothing hotter than inspiration.
- I release myself from the weight of taking a stab at flawlessness.
- I value my body.
- At whatever point I look in the mirror, I always observe something positive.
- I think that it's simple to contemplate my body.
- My body is beautiful, and I regard it profoundly.
- I am thankful for all that my body permits me to do.
- I am thankful for my health.
- I deal with the requirements of my body.
- I acknowledge my body as it is at this moment.
- I appreciate liking my body.
- Discharging Your Negative Emotions About Food
- I release any blame I have about my relationship with food!

- I release any accuse I feel about my relationship with food!
- I release any anger I feel in my relationship with food!
- I release any dread I have in my relationship with food!
- I release any contention I have in my relationship with food!
- I release any cravings I have in my relationship with food!
- I release any sorrow I have in my relationship with food!
- I release any disgrace I feel in my relationship with food!
- I release any sentiments of feebleness I feel in my relationship with food!
- I release any tension I have in my relationship with food!
- I release any longings I have in my relationship with food!
- I release the conviction that a few foods are corrupt!

- I release the conviction that there are correct foods and wrong foods!
- I release ALL the dread based convictions I hold about food!
- I release the conviction that I am a survivor of my digestion!
- I release the conviction that I am a survivor of my qualities!
- I release the conviction that I am helpless before my fat cells!
- I release the conviction that I wouldn't have a sense of security being thin!
- I release the conviction that I am feeble willed!
- I release any sentiments of dismissal I have in my relationship with food!
- I release any dread about unsafe fixings that might be in my food!
- I clear any ways that I despise my body!
- I clear all the clashing feelings I have about food!
- I release and totally let go of all the dread based messages about food and health that I am immersed with consistently!

- I release the habit of utilizing food as a substitute for friendship!
- I release the way I attempt to stuff my sentiments and fill that difficult spot with food!
- I clear all the ways I mistake food for love!
- I release the conviction that my overabundance weight protects me!
- I release the love/detest parts of my relationship with food!
- I release the blame I feel when I eat something experts let me know is terrible for me!
- I release all self-hatred I feel!
- I clear all the ways I stress over my health and weight!
- I release all the ways I hate my body!
- I clear all the ways I don't trust I picked my body!

CHAPTER TWENTY-EIGHT: AFFIRMATIONS TO HEAL YOUR RELATIONSHIP WITH FOOD

Here are 30 affirmations to assist you with settling on healthy food decisions:

Planning Meals

• Planning healthy suppers is a delight.

• Hello, kitchen, you are my sustenance place. I value you!

• I have everything I have to assist me with planning flavorful, nutritious suppers.

• I am so appreciative to pick food that bolsters my best health.

• I can, without much of a stretch, make a nutritious, heavenly dinner.

• I love investing energy in the kitchen!

• I merit the time and cash I put resources into my health.

• I am lucky to the point that I can pick healthy foods for my family.

• My family loves to eat healthy food.

• The kids love to attempt new foods.

• I am learning new things that mend my body with extra special care.

• I will set aside this effort to support myself.

Eating Meals

• I am so thankful for this superb food.

• I am very much sustained in anticipation of the day in front of me.

• My body mends and fortifies with each nibble I take.

• My family assembles with great bliss and love.

• I favor this food and my body with love.

• I tune in for when I am fulfilled and full.

• This food is mending me.

• My taste buds are changing each day-I no longer need foods that don't sustain me.

• I will back off and set aside this effort to feed myself.

General Health

• I emanate certainty, excellence, and beauty.

• Every cell in my body vibrates great health.

• I love and regard my body.

• I pick health and wellbeing over prohibitive diets and disagreeable exercises.

• I feel great when I deal with myself.

• I straightforwardly give and get love.

• Every day I am gotten more grounded and healthier.

• All that I need is within me.

• Every day is another day loaded up with delight and health.

CHAPTER TWENTY-NINE: HOW TO DROP SOME POUNDS FAST

If you're attempting to drop a couple of pounds quickly, these expert tips will make it simple for you to lose weight rapidly.

Include a touch of cushioning number of day by day calories you believe you're eating

If you believe you're devouring 1,700 calories every day and don't comprehend why you're not losing weight, add about another 400 calories to your rough approximation. Examination shows that even dietitians think little of their caloric admission by more than 200 calories, while non-proficient study participants thought little of by 400 calories.

Get an online weight loss amigo to lose more weight

Specialists found that online weight-loss amigos assist you with keeping the weight off. The individuals who included a few companions inside the online weight loss network nearly multiplied the percentage of weight lost contrasted with the individuals who didn't have companions in the program.

Get a weight-loss mantra

You've known about an inevitable outcome? If you continue concentrating on things you can't do, such as opposing junk food or getting out the entryway for a day by day walk, odds are you won't do them. Rather (regardless of whether you in all honesty) repeat positive thoughts to yourself. "I can lose weight." "I will get out for my walk today." "I realize I can oppose the baked good truck after supper." Using contemplation can be another instrument—mindfulness reflection was appeared to help decrease binge eating and passionate significance.

After breakfast, stick to water

At breakfast, feel free to drink a half cup of squeezed orange. Be that as it may, all through the remainder of the day, center around water rather than juice or pop. The average American expends an extra 145 calories every day from soda pops, as indicated by the Centers for Disease Control and Prevention. That is nearly 53,000 calories every year—or 15 pounds! Also, research shows that regardless of the calories, sweet beverages don't trigger a feeling of totality the way that food does.

Eat three fewer nibbles of your feast

Then again, one less treat a day or one less glass of squeezed orange. Doing any of these can spare you around 100 calories every day, and that by itself is sufficient to prevent you from gaining the two pounds many people mindlessly pack on every year. Here are weight loss deceits that have nothing to do with diet or exercise.

Watch one less hour of TV

A study found the more that study participants sat in front of the TV, the more they ate—and the more unhealthy food decisions they made. Sacrifice one program (there's most likely one you would prefer truly not to observe anyway) and take a stroll rather—in even only 15 minutes, you'll receive some astonishing rewards from strolling.

Wash something completely once per week

Regardless of whether that is a story, a few windows, the shower slows down, restroom tile, your vehicle, a 150-pound individual will burn around four calories for consistently spent cleaning. Scour for 30 minutes, and you could work off roughly 120 calories, a similar number in a half-cup of vanilla solidified yogurt.

Hold up until your stomach thunders before you go after food

It's shocking how frequently we eat out of fatigue,

apprehension, habit, or dissatisfaction—so regularly, indeed, that a considerable lot of us have overlooked what physical yearning feels like.

(38 percent of individuals reviewed said they'd eaten unhealthily to manage stress in the previous month.) If you're craving for a specific food, it's most likely a craving, not hunger. If you'd eat anything you could get your hands on, odds are you're genuinely hungry. Figure out how to perceive these sentiments mistaken for hunger; at that point, discover ways other than eating to communicate love, tame stress, and ease fatigue. If you believe you're always ravenous for a clinical explanation, converse with your primary care physician.

Eat before mirrors, and you'll lose weight

One study found that eating before mirrors cut the sum individuals ate by nearly 33%. Looking at yourself without flinching reflects back your very own portion of internal norms and goals and reminds you of why you're attempting to lose weight in any case.

Go through ten minutes a day strolling all over steps

Strolling of any sort is truly an excellent and simple way to lose weight; however, steps, in particular, do some amazing things for weight loss. Examination in the

British Journal of Sports Medicine shows that steps preparing in short blasts, for two to 10 minutes per day, helps lower cholesterol and improve cardiovascular health—permitting you to prepare even more.

Walk five minutes for something like at regular intervals

Stuck at a work area throughout the day? A lively five-minute walk at regular intervals will parlay into an extra 20-minute stroll before the day is over, and getting going is more advantageous than a standing work area. Furthermore, research shows that activity in only five-minute sprays could improve one's health and diminish the danger of death.

You'll lose weight and fat if you walk 45 minutes per day, not 30

Exploration shows that 30 minutes of day by day strolling is sufficient to prevent weight gain in most stationary individuals; however, practice past 30 minutes brings about weight and fat loss. Burning an extra 300 calories per day with three miles of energetic strolling (45 minutes ought to do it) could help you lose 30 pounds in a year without even changing the amount you're eating.

Attempt to maintain a strategic

distance from arranged food

Rundowns sugar, fructose, or corn syrup among the initial four fixings on the mark. You should have the option to discover a lower-sugar rendition of a similar kind of food—particularly foods that regularly contain shrouded sugars, similar to serving of mixed greens dressing or pasta sauce. Additionally, evade partially hydrogenated foods, and search for multiple grams of fiber per 100 calories in all grain items. At last, a short fixing list implies fewer flavor enhancers and void calories. It sounds inconceivable, yet you can figure out how to surrender sugar without missing it.

Put your fork or spoon down between each nibble

At the table, taste water every now and again. Blend your eating with stories for your feasting partner of the entertaining things that occurred during your day. Your cerebrum slacks your stomach by around 20 minutes with regards to satiety (totality) signals. If you eat slowly enough, you'll give your gut microbiome time to alarm your mind that you no longer need food.

Toss out your "fat" garments for good

When you've begun losing weight, discard out or give each garment that doesn't fit, and fill your closet with garments that do. Having to purchase an entirely different closet if you gain the weight back may fill in as a motivation to remain fit.

Close the kitchen for 12 hours

After supper, wash all the dishes, wipe down the counters, kill the light, and, if important, tape closed the cupboards and cooler. Late-evening eating increases the general number of calories you eat, studies found.

Walk directly after supper, and you'll trigger more weight loss

A little study found that strolling directly after you eat can increase weight loss over holding off on a stroll for 60 minutes. Here are quick weight loss tips from nourishment masters.

Make one social excursion this week a functioning one

Pass on the motion pictures and look at the perspectives of a nearby park. Not exclusively will you sit less; however, you'll be sparing calories because you won't chow down on that basin of popcorn. Other dynamic thoughts: a tennis match, a guided nature or city walk, a bicycle ride, and bowling.

Use a stage tracker, and focus on an

extra 1,000 stages every day

It is safe to say that you feel like you have to move more? On average, inactive individuals make just 2,000 to 3,000 strides every day. Including 2,000 stages will assist you with keeping up your present weight and quit gaining weight, including more than that is one of the simple ways to lose weight—and the 10,000 perfect is unquestionably in your range.

Use little plates, and you'll eat little bits

Rather than utilizing standard supper plates that run nowadays from 10 to 14 inches (making them look unfilled if they're not loaded with food), serve your first seminar on little serving of mixed greens plates (around 7 to 9 inches wide). Rather than 16-ounce glasses and curiously large espresso cups, come back to the past times of 8-ounce glasses and 6-ounce espresso cups. That will discourage you from stuffing your plate—and your stomach.

Eat 90 percent of your suppers at home

You're bound to eat more—and eat all the more high-fat, fatty foods—when you eat out than when you eat at home. Eateries today serve such enormous parts that many have changed to bigger plates and tables to suit them. What's more, research shows that food arranged at home is normally healthfully superior to that eatery feast.

Try not to eat with an enormous gathering

A study found that we will, in general, eat more when we eat with others, undoubtedly because we invest more energy at the table. However, eating with your significant other or your family, and utilizing table time for talking in the middle of biting, can help cut down on calories.

Request the littlest part of everything

If you're out and requesting a sub, get the six-inch sandwich. Purchase a little popcorn, a little serving of mixed greens, a little cheeseburger. Again, studies discover we will, in general, eat what's before us, even though we'd feel similarly as full on less.

Eat water-rich foods, and you'll eat fewer calories in general

A body of exploration out of Pennsylvania State University finds that eating water-rich foods, for example, zucchini, tomatoes, and cucumbers during suppers, lessens your general calorie utilization. Other water-rich foods incorporate soups and plates of mixed greens. You won't get similar advantages by simply drinking your water, though (yet you will get different advantages of remaining hydrated). Because the body forms appetite and thirst through different instruments, it just doesn't enlist a feeling of totality with water (or pop, tea, espresso, or juice).

Beef up your suppers with veggies

You can eat twice as much pasta serving of mixed greens stacked with veggies like broccoli, carrots, and tomatoes for indistinguishable calories from a pasta plate of mixed greens donning just mayonnaise. The same goes for sautés, omelets, and other veggie-accommodating dishes. If you eat a 1:1 proportion of grains to veggies, the high-fiber veggies will help fulfill your appetite before you overeat the grains. Reward: Fiber is exceptionally useful for preventing blockage, which can make you look enlarged.

Maintain a strategic distance from white foods

There is some scientific authenticity to today's lower-carb diets: Large measures of refined starches from white flour and included sugar can unleash the destruction of your glucose and lead to weight gain. The breaking points your admission of sugar, white rice, and white flour; trade them for whole-grain breads and earthy colored rice. A few studies have found that eating all the more entire grains makes you bound to weigh less.

Frosted espresso to go. Solidified espresso ice 3D squares in vacuum flagon poured with milk. Hand putting a canteen cover over the jug. White foundation, body parts, individual perspective shot. Detached, duplicate space.

Change to standard espresso

Extravagant espresso drinks from stylish espresso joints frequently pack a few hundred calories, on account of whole milk, whipped cream, sugar, and sweet syrups— and nearly 67 percent of us prefer our espresso with a fatty include ins. Some ordinary espresso with skim milk has only a little portion of those calories. Also, when prepared with great beans, it tastes similarly as great.

Appreciate fatty treats as the highlight, not the focal point

Eating pastry consistently can be beneficial for you, as long as you don't try too hard. Make a spoonful of dessert the gem and a bowl of fruit the crown. Cut down on the chips by blending each nibble with loads of stout, filling new salsa. Offset a little cheddar with a great deal of fruit or plate of mixed greens.

Eat high-fiber grain for breakfast

One study found that individuals who ate oat-or grain-based oats had a lower danger of heftiness contrasted and the individuals who didn't. While individuals who eat fiber-rich grains may have different habits that additionally help prevent weight, those kinds of oat likewise convey more fiber and supplements—and fewer calories—than other breakfast foods. Make oats, or spill out a high-fiber, low-sugar oat like Total or Grape Nuts.

Attempt hot sauce, salsa, and Cajun seasonings

They furnish bunches of flavor with hardly any calories, in addition to they turn up your stomach related flames, making your body briefly burn a couple of more calories. Pick them over margarine and velvety or sweet sauces.

Eat fruit as opposed to drinking fruit juice

For the calories in a single child-size box of squeezed apple, you can appreciate an apple, orange, and a cut of watermelon. These whole foods will keep you fulfilled any longer than that case of squeezed apple, so you'll eat less by and large. Also, research has demonstrated that there's no difference in the effect on your body between drinking fruit juice and drinking pop or other sweet beverage.

Snack on a little bunch of nuts

Studies have found that overweight individuals who ate a moderate-fat diet containing almonds lost more weight than a benchmark group that didn't eat nuts. Snacking on more than one occasion per day is one of the simple ways to lose weight, which helps fight offing yearning and keeps your digestion stirred.

Likewise, you can get together infant carrots or your own path and blend in with the healthiest nuts you can eat, in addition to raisins, seeds, and dried fruit.

Get the greater part of your calories before early afternoon

Studies find that the more you eat in the first part of the day, the less you'll eat in the evening. What's more, you have more chances to burn off those early-day calories than you never really off supper calories.

Brush your teeth after each supper, particularly supper

That perfect, minty newness will fill in as a signal to your body and mind that mealtime is finished. Here are mind stunts to stop enthusiastic eating.

Serve food in courses

Rather than heaping everything on one plate, get food to

the table individual courses. For the initial two courses, bring out soup or veggies, such as a green serving of mixed greens or the most filling fruits and vegetables. When you get to the more calorie-thick foods, similar to meat and treat, you'll be eating less or may as of now be full.

CONCLUSION

It's Weigh-Easy to lose weight with Major Mindset Hypnosis. No resolve required. No medications. No shots. No pills. What's more, the best part about Weigh-Easy is that you eat genuine food every single day. You can even eat frozen yogurt, pizza, pasta and all the solace food you like. No limitations! You will discover that all the foods you love make you full quicker, so you like to eat less of them. Shockingly, you will, in general, crunch on healthy foods and wind up getting a charge out of the water over pop and lager, fruits and veggies over chips and fries, and a lively stroll to the vehicle in lieu of the valet. It's Weigh-Easy to lose weight when your inner mind is ready for your cognizant wants. Lose Weight Hypnosis is for grown-ups and youngsters.

With Major Mindset Hypnosis, the days of eating when stressed are finished! The days of eating because you are annoyed or angry are finished! Presently your weight will no longer mirror your anger and disappointment. For a considerable length of time, poor eating habits conceal stress, misery, dread, and restless sentiments. Through Major Mindset Hypnosis, your subliminal possibly lets you eat when you are ravenous, not when you feel stress, strain, or misery.

Lose Weight Hypnosis! It's "Weigh-Easy" to lose weight. Go profound within your inner mind to change your food viewpoint to begin eating great — as the meager individual who you realize that you are! It's "Weigh-Easy" to lose weight through Major Mindset Hypnosis.

You have settled on the correct decision by getting your copy of this book.

CPSIA information can be obtained
at www.ICGtesting.com
Printed in the USA
BVHW041038231120
593970BV00007B/120